NEPHROLOGY RESEARCH AND CLINICAL DEVELOPMENTS

# ACUTE KIDNEY INJURY

# DETECTION, PREDICTORS AND LONG-TERM OUTCOMES

# NEPHROLOGY RESEARCH AND CLINICAL DEVELOPMENTS

Additional books in this series can be found on Nova's website under the Series tab.

Additional e-books in this series can be found on Nova's website under the e-book tab.

NEPHROLOGY RESEARCH AND CLINICAL DEVELOPMENTS

# ACUTE KIDNEY INJURY

## DETECTION, PREDICTORS AND LONG-TERM OUTCOMES

ERIKA PEARSON
EDITOR

*New York*

Additional color graphics may be available in the e-book version of this book.

**Library of Congress Cataloging-in-Publication Data**

ISBN: 978-1-53610-379-3
Library of Congress Control Number: 2016956155

*Published by Nova Science Publishers, Inc. † New York*

# CONTENTS

# PREFACE

Acute kidney injury (AKI) is a major health concern because it is associated with increased morbidity and mortality. While therapies for AKI have improved in recent years, the prevalence of this condition is still high and continues to increase. Considering these clinical issues, the appropriate detection and management of risk factors related to AKI are important issues for clinicians managing AKI patients. This book discusses the forms of detection, predictors and long-term outcomes for acute kidney injuries.

Chapter 1 - Acute kidney injury (AKI) commonly occurs in hospitalized patients and is independently and strongly associates with morbidity and mortality. The clinical benefits of a timely and definitively diagnosis of AKI have not been fully realized due to limitations imposed by the use of serum Cr and urine output to fulfill diagnostic criteria. These restrictions often lead to diagnostic delays, potential misclassification of actual injury status, and provide little information regarding underlying cause. Novel bio-markers of damage have shown ability to reflect ongoing kidney injury and help further refine existing Risk, Injury, Failure, Loss, End-stage kidney disease (RIFLE) and Acute Kidney injury Network (AKIN) diagnostic criteria. On the basis of published data on the ability of novel damage bio-markers to provide diagnostic and prognostic information on AKI, the authors recommend that novel damage bio-markers may, in the appropriate clinical setting and context (situation consistent with AKI), be used to diagnose AKI even in the absence of changes in Scr or presence of oliguria as described in the existing RIFLE/AKIN criteria for diagnosis of AKI. Adding injury bio-markers as a criteria for AKI will complement the ability of RIFLE/AKIN to define AKI. Promising diagnostic injury markers include neutrophil gelatinase-associated lipocalin (NGAL), kidney injury molecule 1 (KIM-1), interleukin 18 (IL-18) and liver-type fatty acid binding protein (L-FABP).

Several general and setting-specific prediction scores have been developed to identity which patients are at higher risk for AKI following exposure to an acute renal stressor. The most commonly studied clinical settings are cardiac surgery (CABG), iodinated contrast and other nephrotoxin exposure, as well as in the critically ill. However, there are currently insufficient data on damage bio-markers to support their use for AKI staging. Rigorous validation studies measuring the association between the novel damage bio-markers and clinically relevant outcomes are needed.

Patients who develop AKI have worse outcomes characterized by higher mortality, prolonged duration of hospitalization and increased risk for progression to CKD. The severity of AKI predicts progression to CKD and thus there is a clinical need to identify patients who are at a high risk of developing progressive kidney disease, rather than complete recovery from AKI. Bio-markers could help identify risk for in complete recovery and long-term progression to CKD and allow the earlier introduction of conventional or even novel interventional therapy.

Chapter 2 - New biomarkers for acute kidney injury (AKI) have been proposed; however, they require further validation for use in routine clinical practice. Older biomarkers that are commonly monitored for other purposes have shown potential for predicting the risk of AKI. Complete blood counts (e.g., white blood cells and their subtypes, hemoglobin, red cell distribution width, and platelet volume) are known to be predictors for AKI; however, the natures of the relationships are different for each marker and may be U-shaped, linear, and non-linear with a threshold level. An electrolyte panel (e.g., sodium, potassium, and bicarbonate) is also predictive of AKI, even though the causal relationship is not validated. The baseline liver panel (e.g., liver enzymes, bilirubin, and albumin) strongly predicts subsequent development of AKI, particularly in patients with liver disease or where the liver has been manipulated. Proteinuria and hematuria are easily measured using the dipstick test and are representative markers of chronic kidney injury. They are also predictors for AKI, although the test's low precision and misclassification bias should be acknowledged. Considering these results, this review suggests that old biomarkers can be interpreted for additional clinical usefulness in the prediction of AKI.

Chapter 3 - Acute kidney injury (AKI) is common in clinical settings and an independent predictor of mortality in critically ill patients.

Thus, prevention and early detection of compromised renal function based on serum creatinine levels, urinary output and urinary/serum biomarkers are routinely used in clinical practice. However, appropriate antibiotic treatment is the best lifesaving option in almost all cases of sepsis. Antibiotic treatment is of paramount importance in critically ill septic patients with/without renal damage but a major problem is the necessity for antibiotic drugs with known nephrotoxicity and effects on renal function. In patients with renal replacement and consequently altered antibiotic elimination dynamics, this is of particular relevance. On the other hand, of antibiotic efficacy is reduced if the treatment is not sufficiently controlled. Therapeutic drug monitoring is the most appropriate method for treating septic patients with AKI and for optimising antimicrobial drug serum concentrations without worsening renal function.

In: Acute Kidney Injury
Editor: Erika Pearson
ISBN: 978-1-53610-379-3


*Chapter 1*

# USE BIOMARKERS OF ACUTE KIDNEY INJURY TO DETECT, PREDICT, AND ASSESS PROGNOSIS

***Shutian Xu**[*] **and Zheng Tang***
National Clinical Research Center of Kidney Diseases,
Jinling Hospital Nanjing University School of Medicine

## ABSTRACT

Acute kidney injury (AKI) commonly occurs in hospitalized patients and is independently and strongly associates with morbidity and mortality. The clinical benefits of a timely and definitively diagnosis of AKI have not been fully realized due to limitations imposed by the use of serum Cr and urine output to fulfill diagnostic criteria. These restrictions often lead to diagnostic delays, potential misclassification of actual injury status, and provide little information regarding underlying cause. Novel bio-markers of damage have shown ability to reflect ongoing kidney injury and help further refine existing Risk, Injury, Failure, Loss, End-stage kidney disease (RIFLE) and Acute Kidney injury Network (AKIN) diagnostic criteria. On the basis of published data on the ability of novel damage bio-markers to provide diagnostic and prognostic information on AKI, we recommend that novel damage bio-markers may, in the appropriate clinical setting and context (situation consistent with AKI), be used to diagnose AKI even in the absence of changes in Scr or presence

[*] Corresponding author: tinne_xst@163.com.

of oliguria as described in the existing RIFLE/AKIN criteria for diagnosis of AKI. Adding injury bio-markers as a criteria for AKI will complement the ability of RIFLE/AKIN to define AKI. Promising diagnostic injury markers include neutrophil gelatinase-associated lipocalin (NGAL), kidney injury molecule 1 (KIM-1), interleukin 18 (IL-18) and liver-type fatty acid binding protein (L-FABP).

Several general and setting-specific prediction scores have been developed to identity which patients are at higher risk for AKI following exposure to an acute renal stressor. The most commonly studied clinical settings are cardiac surgery (CABG), iodinated contrast and other nephrotoxin exposure, as well as in the critically ill. However, there are currently insufficient data on damage bio-markers to support their use for AKI staging. Rigorous validation studies measuring the association between the novel damage bio-markers and clinically relevant outcomes are needed.

Patients who develop AKI have worse outcomes characterized by higher mortality, prolonged duration of hospitalization and increased risk for progression to CKD. The severity of AKI predicts progression to CKD and thus there is a clinical need to identify patients who are at a high risk of developing progressive kidney disease, rather than complete recovery from AKI. Bio-markers could help identify risk for in complete recovery and long-term progression to CKD and allow the earlier introduction of conventional or even novel interventional therapy.

## AKI DETECTION

Acute kidney injury (AKI) is increasingly recognized as an in hospital complication that is common and strongly related to increased hospital length of stay, use of intensive care unit services including hemodynamic monitoring, need for renal replacement therapy, rehospitalization, and death. When patients are followed after an episode of AKI, there are higher risks for the rapid progression of chronic kidney disease leading to end-stage renal disease requiring permanent dialysis therapy or renal transplantation. Hence, there is a great need to better understand AKI with the intent of developing prevention and treatment strategies. Prior to the past few years, the principle clinical tools used to detect AKI were serial measurement of serum Cr, blood urea nitrogen (BUN), assessment of the urinalysis, and measurement of urine output (UO). Agreement from multiple consensus groups (Acute kidney Injury Network-AKIN, Risk, Injury, Failure, End-stage Kidney Disease-RIFLE, and Kidney Disease Improving Global Outcomes-KDIGO) that AKI can be defined and graded has been a major advance in phenotypic characterization as shown in

Figure 1 [1]. Thus the stage has been set for new technologies and measures to be assessed in the context of both the diagnosis and grading of AKI according to these standardized definitions [2].

## DIAGNOSIS OF AKI

The diagnosis of AKI using the AKIN (Acute Kidney Injury Network) or RIFLE criteria is currently limited as Cr and UO can only indirectly reflect that kidney damage has occurred. These criteria, by definition, are retrospective in nature an require at least 6h to several days, thus inherently delaying the clinical diagnosis of AKI [3, 4]. The UO criteria for AKI diagnosis (<0.5ml/kg/h for > 6h) are hindered by limited sensitivity when diuretics are administered, reduced specificity in the presence of dehydration, and lack of practicality in measurement when an indwelling urinary catheter is not present [5]. These limitations have contributed to the inability to successfully characterize various aspects of the disease, consistently identify individuals at risk, and translate promising preclinical therapeutic strategies into successful treatments.

**RIFLE criteria (within 7 days)**

| Class | GFR criteria | Urine output criteria |
|---|---|---|
| R-Risk | Creatinine increase × 1.5 or GFR loss > 25% | 0.5 < mL/kg/hour × >6 hours |
| I-Injury | Creatinine increase × 2 or GFR loss > 50% | 0.5 < mL/kg/hour × >12 hours |
| F-Failure | Creatinine increase × 3 or GFR loss > 75% or creatinine increase >4 mg/dL (acute increase >0.5 mg/dL) | 0.3 < mL/kg/hour × >24 hours or anuria >12 hours |
| L-Loss | Persistent loss of kidney function >4 weeks | |
| E-ESKD | ESKD > 3 months | |

**AKIN criteria (within 48 hours)**

| Stage | Serum creatinine criteria | Urine output criteria |
|---|---|---|
| 1 | Creatinine increase × 1.5 or creatinine increase >0.3 mg/dL | 0.5 < mL/kg/hour × >6 hours |
| 2 | Creatinine increase × 2 | 0.5 < mL/kg/hour × >12 hours |
| 3 | Creatinine increase × 3 or creatinine increase >4 mg/dL (acute increase >0.5 mg/dL) | 0.3 < mL/kg/hour × >24 hours or anuria >12 hours |

Figure 1. The AKIN and RIFILE definitions and grading for AKI. Patients who receive renal replacement therapy (RRT) are considered to have met the criteria for stage 3 irrespective of the stage that they are in at the time of commencement of RRT.

As shown in Figure 2, the combination of simultaneous assessment of a functional and damage markers can help stratify patients into 4 subgroups: no marker change, functional alone, damage alone, or change in both functional and damage markers. This categorization permits identification of a new category of patients who may have 'subclinical' AKI, i.e., an increase in damage markers without a simultaneous loss of kidney function (Figure 2, upper right quadrant). In these conditions, e.g., nephrotoxic drug exposure, loss of function may not develop at all or be seen at some time interval after detection of renal injury. Although direct evidence is sparse, it appears that these patients are at higher risk for adverse outcomes including need for RRT and mortality, than patients without an increase in damage biomarker levels [6].

| | No damage | Damage present |
|---|---|---|
| No functional change | No functional changes or damage | Damage without loss of function |
| Functional change | Loss of function without damage | Damage with loss of function |

Figure 2. New spectrum of AKI based on combination of functional and damage bio-markers.

## EARLY DETECTION OF ACUTE KIDNEY INJURY

The first ADQI workgroup focused on the available literature on novel blood and urine bio-markers that have been tested in clinical studies for the early detection of AKI. Recognition that cells in the kidney produce and release measurable proteins in the setting of a variety of injuries has been an important step in the development of this field [7]. Injury appears to be as subtle as volume depletion which has been previously termed “prerenal azotemia”. Data with novel markers suggest these episodes are indeed a form of AKI with some damage to cells and complete nephron units [8]. More severe causes of renal damage include prolonged ischemia due to shock, sepsis and microcirculatory of dysfunction, and direct toxicity due to injurious agents such as iodinated contrast, aminoglycosides, and vancomycin. Most of the markers mentioned in the accompanying article by McCullough and colleagues are either directly produced by renal tubular cells in response to upregulation of messenger RNA and RNA and protein synthesis, or are filtered proteins that have reduced reabsorption by the proximal tubular cells, and hence become measurable in greater quantities in the urine. Tubular cell-cycle arrest markers (insulin-like growth factor-binding protein 7(IGFBP7) and tissue inhibitor of metalloproteinases-2(TIMP-2) appear to be a brief (-36h) harbinger to AKI that will develop in the new days [9]. The concentrations of these proteins in the urine can be multiplied to create a value for use by clinicians to anticipate the immediate risk of AKI. The development of AKI from initiation of injury forward appears to be reflected by sharp elevation of neutrophil gelatinase-associated lipocalin (NGAL), kidney injury molecule-1(KIM-1), L-type fatty acid-binding protein (L-FABP), and α-glutathione S-transferase (α-GST), [illegible]-GST, and interleukin-18 (IL-18). The preponderance of the data suggests these novel markers detect risk for AKI and probably actual AKI 24-48h before the rise in serum Cr [10]. Importantly, there are cases where novel markers significantly elevate without a significant change in serum Cr or reduction in UO, which is a late and ominous clinical development [11]. These cases of subclinical AKI appear to have important prognostic implications and probably should not to be dismissed (Figure 3).

Based on this new conceptual framework, we recommend a modification of the AKIN/RIFLE criteria to incorporate the use of kidney damage markers in addition to Scr, GFR and UO (Figure 3). Under this new diagnostic approach, in the appropriate clinical setting, AKI can be defined by abnormal levels of kidney injury bio-markers even in the absence of oliguria or elevated Scr. The bulk of evidence has focused on the following damage bio-markers including urinary/plasma NGAL, urinary KIM-1, urinary IL-18, and L-FABP. Several additional markers are in development and may also become commercially available over the short term. Most of these studies have focused on determining the time course of change in the biomarker in relation to a change in Scr. However, the timing of biomarker assessment has not been concurrent with Scr or UO assessment thereby introducing an inherent bias favoring the bio-markers. Nevertheless, the time course of the biomarker change preceding any functional change suggests that it should be feasible to identify patients at a point in the course where they only have alteration in the injury markers.

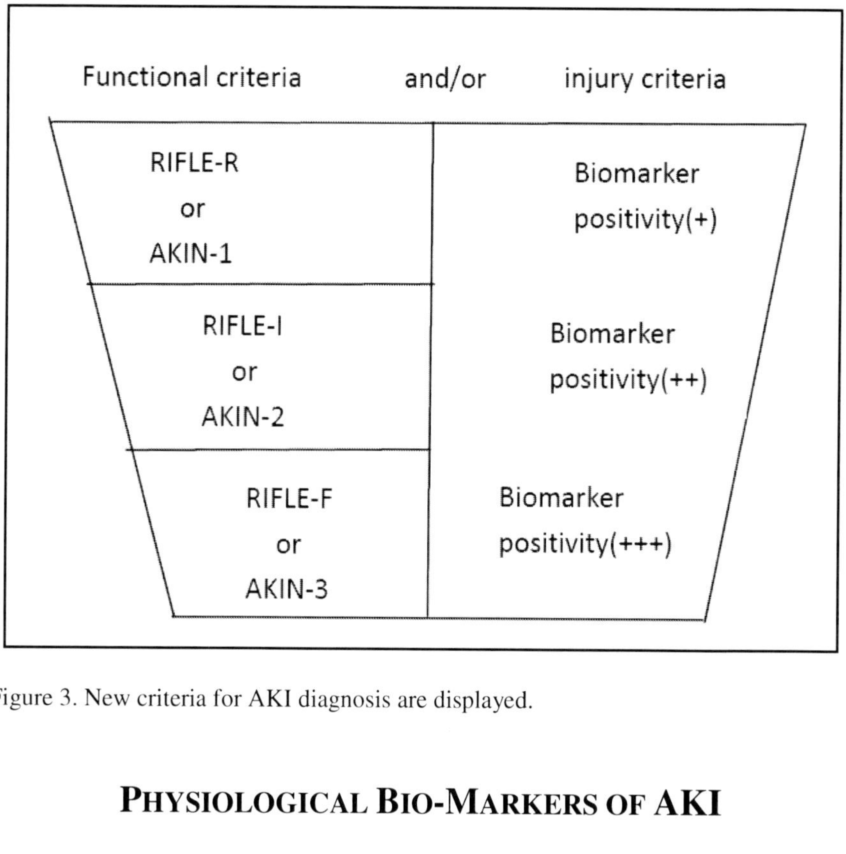


Figure 3. New criteria for AKI diagnosis are displayed.

## PHYSIOLOGICAL BIO-MARKERS OF AKI

The discovery and validation of novel bio-markers of kidney damage over the past decade represent major advances in the field of AKI. The investment by major sponsors and investigators demonstrates a consensus that early bio-markers of AKI are needed. These damage bio-markers proved to be sensitive and specific in a number of small clinical studies. Damage bio-markers are biochemical markers of early cellular injury that can be measured upon release from cells into the plasma or urine. However, long before ischemic cellular injury alterations in the renal microcirculation and tissue oxygenation occur, rendering epithelial cells susceptible to injury. These pathophysiological processes represent microcirculatory dysfunction ultimately leading to AKI. In addition, renal auto regulatory mechanisms are invoked in response to renal insults and play an important role in maintaining homeostasis. The underlying state of health of the kidney and the effective ‘renal reserve’ are important determinants of this auto regulatory response to modify renal function in response to injury. Currently, our ability to detect these changes in kidney function or structure has been limited to measurement of UO and changes in serum Cr reflecting alterations in the glomerular filtration rate (GFR). These measurements represent the physiological bio-markers to track the development and course of AKI and are the current parameters utilized for diagnosis and staging of AKI. However, several additional tools are now available to ascertain physiological response to kidney injury. Couple with the emerging damage markers, these physiological bio-markers might help identify patients at risk, and provide mechanistic information and a window for therapeutic intervention to prevent AKI. As an example, we have developed a modified description of the clinical phases of ischemic AKI [12] that incorporates physiological parameters that complement the use of biochemical bio-markers and clinical characteristics for the study of AKI (Figure 4).

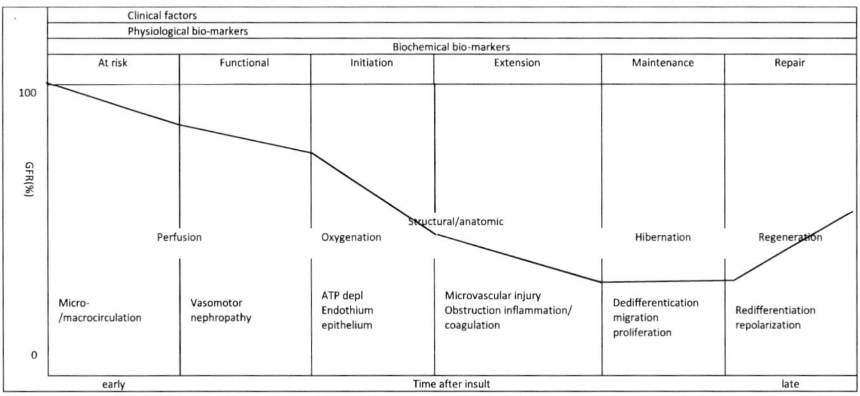


Figure 4. Physiological phases of AKI following ischemia-reperfusion injury.

# Renal Blood Flow, Tissue Oxygenation and Microcirculatory Function: Critical Physiological Bio-Markers

Adequate parenchymal oxygen is an essential physiological requirement for sustaining kidney cell viability. In the kidney, 90% of oxygen consumption sustains oxidative phosphorylation for ATP production and sodium reabsorption [13]. Since sodium reabsorption is intrinsically dependent on sodium load, renal oxygen consumption is in turn highly dependent on the GFR and renal blood flow (RBF) [14]. RBF, blood flow distribution between cortex and medulla and microcirculatory blood flow may change prior to changes in damage bio-markers and may serve as one of the earliest indicators of altered renal function and complement damage bio-markers. Hyperfiltration and an increase in RBF [15] may reflect differences in 'renal reserve' and assessment of this parameter may provide information on risk of AKI. Autoregulation maintains normal GFR and RBF when mean arterial pressures drop to ~80mmHg. This is accomplished through a decrease in afferent arteriolar tone mediated by vasodilators such as prostaglandins and increase in efferent arteriolar tone mediated by angiotension II. Prior to tubular injury, alterations in RBF may represent the earliest measureable physiological changes. In the absence of adequate oxygen supply, the kidney is at risk for failure [16]. Pathological processes such as AKI disrupt the balance between tissue oxygen, nitric oxide and radical oxygen species [17].

Existing and developing non-invasive techniques to measure physiological parameters of kidney function in AKI are listed in Table 1. The known clinical characteristics of each of these techniques are included in Table 2. For example, contrast-enhanced ultrasound (CEU) may be used to determine 'renal reserve' by measuring changes in RBF in response to a protein load [18]. This maneuver could potentially identify subjects who lack reserve capacity and may be at higher risk for AKI. Near infrared spectroscopy or blood oxygenation level-dependent (BOLD) magnetic resonance imaging (MRI) may be used for detection of changes in oxygenation of the kidney. Detection of changes in oxygenation could identify those individuals at risk for AKI.

**Table 1. Physiological bio-markers for assessment of kidney function in AKI**

| |
|---|
| Glomerular filtration rate/urine flow monitoring |
| • Urine indices |
| • Real-time GFR measurement |
| • Serial serum creatinine measurement (with correction for fluid balance using bioelectrical impedance analysis) |
| • continuous urine flow |
| Renal perfusion |
| • Doppler ultrasound (visualization of macrocirculation) |
| • Contrast-enhanced ultrasound (visualization of microcirculation) |
| Renal oxygenation |
| • Bladder tissue pO2 |
| • Bladder urine pO2 (measure of renal O2 bioavailability) |
| • Near infrared spectroscopy (measure of renal O2 bioavailability) |
| • Bold MRI (measure of renal metabolism) |
| Other complimentary markers |
| • kidney ultrasound |
| • Renal venous O2 saturation (measurement of renal oxygen consumption) |
| • Urinalysis (renal indices, urine sediment, flow cytometry) |
| • Endothelial markers (e.g., Endothelial microparticles, glycocalyx degradation) |
| • Inflammatory markers (e.g., Cytokines, immune cells) |
| • Oxidative stress markers |

## Glomerular Filtration Rate, Continuous Urine Output Measurement, and Urine Indices

### Real-Time GFR Measurement

Determination of GFR is of utmost importance for evaluating kidney function in patients with kidney disease and for appropriate drug dosing. The clearance of an ideal filtration marker such as inulin, iothalamate or iohexol, is the gold standard for measuring GFR [19]. However, these cumbersome, time-consuming techniques are not practical for use in clinical practice. A transcutaneous remote real-time analysis of FITC-sinistrin excretion has been used to determine GFR in healthy rats and rat with kidney disease [20]. In these studies, comparative measurements of transcutaneous and plasma elimination kinetics of FITC-sinistrin were compared, and highly comparable GFR values were demonstrated in all animal groups.

Lately, a point-of-care bedside fluorescence-based measured GFR (mGFR) assay has been developed experimentally for the rapid measurement of GFR [20, 21], which has potential applicability in AKI. In the main descriptive study, fluorescent conjugates of a small freely filterable reporter (inulin) and a large non-filterable marker (500kDa dextan) were infused as a bolus, and the *in vivo* fluorescent signals were detected and quantified by the ratiometric optical fiber system [21]. The plasma volume was estimated by dilution of the large dextran molecule and the GFR was determined using the ratiometric two-compartment method 60 min after the injection. This method presented excellent agreement with the concurrent 6-hour iohexol-based GFR measurement technique.

In summary, fully developed real-time transcutaneous or intravascular monitoring of GFR may prove to be an ideal bedside tool for risk stratification, early diagnosis, prognosis and therapy guidance in AKI.

## Serial Creatinine Measurement

Serum Cr is an inexpensive and readily available physiological biomarker of kidney function and remain the 'gold standard' test for diagnosing AKI [22, 23], however it is non-specific for the nature and extent of injury and is influenced by several factors including the volume of distribution requiring adjustments for the levels of fluid accumulation (prior to) achievement of steady-state conditions) [24]. For these reasons, it is considered a suboptimal GFR marker [25] and a late biomarker of AKI when both damage and physiological change occur together. More frequent measurements might allow earlier detection of AKI and could provide valuable insight into the mechanism and pathways to track the course of AKI. This hypothesis need to be formally tested.

## Continuous Urine Output Measurement

The importance of urine output in the detection of AKI has recently been preliminarily verified [26], providing support for continuously monitoring urine output. A recent study assessed the use of an electronic urine output monitoring device in 20 critically ill patients [27]. Urine volume was measured using a drip detector, based on infrared detection. In this study, hourly urine output was measured with both traditional urinometer and continuous urine output monitoring device; both validated by cylinder measurements. Positive predictive value for AKI of a urine output of 40ml/h was 91% with the continuous urine output monitoring device, and 77% with the urinometer. Additional studies are needed to further validate the performance of this user-friendly system and to prospectively evaluate whether urine output combined with serial Cr measurements provide reliable, robust predictive tools in the setting of AKI.

### Fractional Excreting of Sodium and Urea, and Urine Osmolality

Urine sodium and osmolality have been standard urine indices used in differentiating pre-renal AKI from acute tubular necrosis for decades. In a small study of patients with various forms of AKI, the fractional excretion of sodium (FeNa) proved to be useful. Although FeNa correctly diagnosed 86 of 87 patients, and urinary osmolality and urinary sodium correctly diagnosed AKI in 46 and 60% of patients, respectively [28], numerous exceptions limit the value of these clinical tests [29].

The measurement of the fractional excretion of urea (Feurea) may be useful in patients with AKI. Studies have documented an Feurea of 50-60% in patients with acute tubular necrosis compared to values below 35% in patient with pre-renal AKI. Although this urine index may be more useful than Feurea in patients who have received diuretics, it should not be used in isolation [30]. The traditional use of FeNa and Feurea will need to be reconsidered given the growing concept that pure functional loss may also be associated with damage and altered tubular function. For example, we will need to understand the dianostic and prognostic significance of FeNa and Feurea of <1% and 35%, respectively, when damage bio-markers are positive.

## ASSESSMENT OF RENAL TISSUE PERFUSION

### Doppler Ultrasound

Using 2D ultrasonography and colour Doppler, systolic and diastolic velocities of interlobar arteries can be measured. The Doppler resistive index (RI) described by Pourcelot ((peak systolic velocity-end diastolic velocity)/peak systolic velocity) is the traditional index used as a measurement of renal vascular resistance. A value of 0.60 is considered to be a normal value for renal RI, whereas 0.7 is usually cosidered to be the upper threshold of normal RI in adult [31]. This index has been proposed for the quantification of the changes in renal vascular resistance but may be affected by other factors such as central hemodynamics (especially artery stiffness, pulse pressure and heart rate), interstitial renal pressure, intra-abdominal pressure and other factors including age and underlying kidney disease. The RI has been found to reflect the degree of parenchymal damage in chronic kidney disease [32, 33] or hypertension [34], predict long-term kidney function in transplanted patients [35] and the diagosis of obstuctive uropathy [36].

Renal Doppler ultrasound has been used to predict AKI [37, 38]. In 37 critically patients with septic shock, the RI predicted the development of AKI 5 days after presentation (RI of 0.77 vs. 0.68 in AKI vs. Non-AKI, respectively) [37]. These findings were recently confirmed in mechanically ventilated patients [38]. The RI was found to be higher in patients with acute tubular necrosis (0.85) than in pre-renal AKI (0.67), and better than urinary indices in the diagnosis of persistent AKI [39]. Finally, the RI might be useful in the assessment of renal circulation during the initial resuscitation in sepsis [40]. These studies indicate that Doppler is a simple, non-invasive tool that may be of significant utility in the setting of AKI (Table 2).

**Table 2. Utility of physiological bio-markers in AKI**

| Physiological biomarker | Risk assessment | Early diagnosis | Different diagnosis | Prognosis | Therapy guidance |
|---|---|---|---|---|---|
| Urine indices | - | √ | √ | - | √ |
| Serial serum creatinine | √ | √ | √ | √ | √ |
| Real-time measured GFR | √ | √ | √ | √ | √ |
| Continuous urine flow | √ | √ | √ | √ | ? |
| Doppler ultrasound | √ | √ | √ | ? | √ |
| Contrast-enhanced ultrasound | √ | √ | √ | ? | √ |
| Urine pO2 | √ | √ | ? | ? | √ |
| Bladder pO2 | √ | | √ | ? | √ |
| BOLD MRI | ? | ? | √ | √ | ? |
| Positron emission tomography | ? | ? | √ | √ | ? |
| Near infrared spectroscopy | ? | ? | √ | √ | ? |
| Bioelectrical impedance analysis | - | √ | - | √ | √ |

## Contrast-Enhanced Ultrasound

The gold standard measurement of RBF is p-aminohippurtate (PAH) clearance. Although relatively accurate, the method has the disadvantage of being time-consuming and expensive. Furthermore, decreased renal tubular extraction in AKI and other high-risk settings (cardiopulmonary bypass, critical illness) largely invalidates this method of RBF measurement in such patients.

Contrast-enhanced ultrasonograhpy, although relatively new in assessing renal echocardiography. Contrast agents used for ultrasonography are gas-filled microbublbles (1-6um in diameter) which scatter ultrasound very effectively and are coated with a protein, lipid or polymer layer [41]. Second-generation microbubbles use inert, poorly soluble perfluorinated gases stablized by phopholipids or albumin [41]. The small size allows microbubbles to provide information on small capillary beds. Although CEU has been used safely in human, there are few studies on its use in AKI. In healthy volunteers, use of drugs to block the renin-angiotensin system produced measurable changes in microbubble perfusion indices that correlated with PAH clearance [42]. CEU has been usedto diagnose renal artery stenosis, and was found to be more sensitive and specific in comparision to color Doppler ultrasound and similar to angiography [43]. In healthy volunteers, CEU detected a 43% increase in RBF following a high protein meal [18]. The ability to determine renal reserve could be useful in identifying patients who are at risk for AKI. Lastly, in kidney transplantation, CEU has been used to identify perfusion abnormalities helpful in the diagnosis of acute rejection [44] and chronic allograft nephropathy [45].

## Bioelectrical Impedance Analysis (BIA)

BIA is a safe non-invasive, rapid and inexpensive technique to measure fluid compartment volume. It measures electrical properties of the body by measuring resistance, reactance and phase angle [46]. This method has been used in assessment nutritional status, urea distribution or dry weight during dialysis. It also has been used to assess intradialytic hypotension, as well as in AKI during CRRT. The use of BIA with serum Cr is supported by recent data suggesting that further accuracy can be gained if serum Cr is corrected for fluid accumulation [24]. The current method to assess fluid accumulation is through daily assessment of fluid balance. The use of BIA can give accurate assessment of total body water within minutes and can provide rapid correction of serum Cr.

# Assessment of Kidney Oxygenation and Metabolism

## Positron Emission Tomography (PET)

PET is an imaging technique that produces three-dimensional images of physiological activity in the body, by detection of pairs of gamma rays emitted by a positron-emitting radinuclide tracer. The tracer is administered on a biologically active molecule, which tracks to specific areas of physiological activity an quantifies processes of biological importance, in an antomical context. In the context of the kidney, PET scanning provides the ability to non-invasively quantify both RBF and kidney metabolism. PET measurement of RBF using 15O-labeled water (H215O) has been validated using radiolabelled microspheres in pigs [47]. Similar analyses in humans with and without kidney disease demonstrate that PET with H215O provides a non-invasive method for quantitative mapping of RBF [48]. PET imaging has also been used to evaluate kidney metabolism. In one such study, PET with 18F-flurodeoxyglucose was used to assess acute rejection in a rat renal transplantation model [49]. Further prospective studies are needed to determine the utility of PET scanning as a tool in the setting of AKI.

## Optical Spectroscopy

Optical Spectroscopy provides a non-invasive method of determining the oxygenation of blood in tissues. Optical spectroscopy uses differing optical absorbance of light in the near infrared (NIR) region (650-900nm) between oxy- and deoxyhemoglobin to assess the oxygenation status in various vascular compartments. NIR spectroscopy devices entail an emitting light source directing light into tissues, and one or more sensors placed cutaneously measuring the returned light at several wavelengths. Currently, NIR spectroscopy devices for monitoring the kidney have only been used in children due to the relative accessibility of the pediatric kidney to NIR light in comparison to that in adults. NIR spectroscopy was first used to non-invasively monitor kidney oxygenation transcutaneously in mechanically ventilated children [50]. The study was able to monitor the effects of spontaneous episodes of oxygen desaturation on the kidney and determine the renal oxygen extraction during these episodes. Another study of NIR spectroscopy in children with heart failure was able to demonstrate a strong correlation between renal NIR spectroscopy values measured at the flank and renal vein saturation [51]. NIR spectroscopy has been used to demonstrate the ability of blood transfusion to effectively oxygenate the kidney in anemic children [52]. This use is of special importance due to the sensitivity of the kidney to hypoxemia and anemia [16]. A study in children undergoing cardiac surgery demonstrated a strong correlation between the low kidney oxygen saturation level and the development of AKI [53].

Direct access to the kidney could provide more direct and detailed measurements. Direct observation of the human renal microcirculation for this purpose has been accomplished by the use of hand-held microscopes [54]. Direct NIR spectroscopy measurement for assessment of renal cortex microcirculatory oxygenation has been combined with a miniature laser Doppler devices to measure microcirculatory oxygenation and perfusion of the kidney cortex for assessing the success of transplantation [55]. Although the current applications are still sparse, it is expected that technical improvements will permit a comprehensive assessment of renal perfusion and oxygenation and provide a robust clinical platform to monitor the progress, response to therapy and resolution of AKI at the bedside.

## BOLD MRI

BOLD MRI is a rapid non-invasive method for assessing renal tissue oxygen bioavailability, relying on the paramagnetic properties of deoxyhemoglobin [56]. The concentration of deoxyhemoglobin increase with rising oxygen consumption, leading to a decreasing T2 relaxation time of the surrounding tissue. Increased R2 (the rate of spin dephasing; equal to 1/T2 relaxation time) levels therefore imply increased deoxyhemoglobin (decreased oxyhemoglobin) and decreased partial pressures of oxygen (PaO2) in renal tissues [56]. The capability of BOLD MRI to evaluate parenchymal oxygen bioavailability in many renal settings has been reported both experimentally and clinically [57-61]. There are fewer studies utilizing BOLD MRI in AKI [62], in acute rejection compared to kidney transplant recipients with prerenal azotemia or acute tubular necrosis [63].

## Urine Oxygen ($O_2$) Tension

O2 tension is the local partial pressure of O2 in the urine (PuO2). The pO2 of urine entering the calyces reflects oxygen tension of the renal medulla, and is determined by O2 supply, renal medullary blood flow, and oxygen consumption and may be the most reliable quantitative index of renal medullary perfusion.

Real-time PuO2 has been measured in anesthetized dogs using the polarographic method [64], which is costly and cumbersome. A newer more promising and less expensive dynamic fluorescence quenching method relies on the collision of an O2 molecule with a fluorophore in its exited state, which leads to a nonradiative transfer of energy [64]. MRI has been used to quantify PuO2 [65].

In studies of anesthetized human voluteers [66], the PuO2 is fair constant under normal conditions. The PuO2 decreases in states of volume depletion and increases following volume re-expansion. In hemorrhagic shock, there is a sharp decline in PuO2. Bladder PuO2 has been measured in settings of critical illness [67], cardiac arrest [66], cardiogenic shock [66], and following onpump cardiac surgery [68], and has been shown to improve by the use of manitol [66] and fenoldopam [67]. In a study of 90 patients undergoing cardiapulmonary bypass surgery, the postoperative serum Cr level was significantly higher in patients whose PuO2 decreased after surgery, as compared with those whose PuO2 remained constant or increased [68]. This study presents the possibility of using bladder PuO2 monitoring for the early detection of postoperative AKI.

## Conclusion

The emergence of novel markers of kidney function offers the promise to provide clinicians with a set of tools to efficiently and more accurately assess the underlying processes result from kidney injury and determine the course and time point for intervention. The choice of physiological biomarker for diagnosis and staging, differential diagnosis, and prognosis of AKI will need to be determined in prospective studies. We believe that an expanded tool kit of physiological bio-markers might significantly enhance our capabilities to recognized AKI early, and provide a better understanding of the pathophysiology of this heterogeneous condition.

# AKI PREDICTION

## Risk Assessment

The risk for developing AKI is based on the cumulative effect of premorbid factors (e.g., comorbidities) that increase susceptibility to kidney damage and reduced function, and the type and severity of intercurrent processs (i.e., stressors) that impact the kidney (Table 3). Several general and setting-specific prediction scores have been developed to identity which patients are at higher risk for AKI following exposure to an acute renal stressor. The most commonly studied clinical settings are cardiac surgery (CABG), iodinated contrast and other nephrotoxin exposure, as well as in the critically ill. In most instances, the emerging bio-markers have not been assessed to predict suceptibility to AKI and are not incorporated in the scores.

**Table 3. Recongnized risk factors and stressors for developing AKI adapted from Goldstein and Chawla [75]**

| Comorbidity | Kidney stressor |
|---|---|
| Age >65 years | Sepsis/shock/hypoxiemia |
| Diabetes mellitus | Volume depletion |
| Cirrhosis/hepatic failure | Cardiopulmonary bypass |
| Heart failure | Exposure to nephrotoxins (e.g., Vancomycin, gentamicin, NSAID, ACEI, ARB, cisplatin/carboplatin, methotrexate) |
| Chronic kidney disease (eGFR< 60ml/min/1.73m2) | Iodinated contrast |
| Albuminuria | Invasive mechanical ventilation |
| Glomerular diseases | Multipleorgan failure |
| Renal transplant recipients | |
| Protein/calorie malnutrition | |

eGFR = estimated glomerular filtration rate; NSAID = nonsteroidal anti-inflammatory agent; ACEI = angiotensin converting enzyme inhibitor; ARB = angiotensin receptor blocker.

While risk assessment scores often perform well during development, few, if any, have demonstrated sufficient ability to be used clinically when generalized to external settings. Individualized risk prediction or early diagnosis is currently not possible from our review of the literature. Even when development-associate variables such as reduced kidney mass at birth and polymorphisms affecting the sympathetic and renin-angiotensin systems are included, accurate prediction is still not possible [69-73]. The most commonly studied clinical settings for AKI risk prediction are timed injury models (cardiac surgery, iodinated contrast exposure, other nephrotoxic agents) and untimed injury scenarios including critical illness with or without sepsis. These are briefly summarized in Table 3.

## Cardiac Surgery

Three risk prediction scores have been recently reviewed and found to have an area under the receiver-operating characteristic curve (AROC) for renal replacement therapy (RRT) of roughly 0.79 [75]. These three scoring systems were not reproducible in other centers, were not suitable for estimation of the true incidence of postoperative need for RRT, were poorly calibrated and tended to underestimate the actual need for RRT [76]. These results are consistent with those from a prior study from the Mayo Clinic [77]. Many scores have not included timing of coronary angiography using iodianted contrast prior to CABG, which is an important determinant of AKI after the operation [78]. Other shortcomings included the use of intraoperative variables and variables that represent complications in the clinical course or are proxies for the baseline severity of illness.

A consistent body of evidence spanning from ischemia/reperfusion-based animal experiments and numerous clinical studies linking damage bio-markers with AKI and adverse patient outcomes following cardiac surgery underlines their diagnostic value with the largest cumulative pediatric and adult patient cohort investigated using NGAL [79, 80]

Injury bio-markers for early diagnosis of AKI were investigated in more than 3,000 cardiac surgical patients with an AKI incidence of ~20% and have been show to rise early, i.e., 2-12h after surgery. The TRIBE (Translational Research Involving bio-markers and Endpoints) study evaluated 1,219 adults undergoing cardiac surgery and reported that urine IL-18 and urine and plasma NGAL levels peaked within 6h after surgery [79]. A clinical prediction model for AKI had an AROC of 0.69. Urine IL-18 and plasma NGAL significantly improved the AROC to 0.76 and 0.75, respectively. Urine IL-18 and plasma NGAL significantly improved risk prediction over the clinical models alone. The TRIBE investigators also evaluated 311 children undergoing surgery for congenital cardiac lesions using the same bio-markers. Similarly, they found that the novel damage markers rose within 6h of surgery and that the AROC improved with urine IL-18 and urine NGAL, but not with plasma NGAL [81]. Thus, we believe novel markers in conjunction with the clinical evaluation and

Cr can be used to diagnose AKI after cardiac surgery, in some cases before obvious renal failure becomes evident.

## Inodinated Contrast Exposure

The best developed prediction scores for contrast-induced AKI (CI-AKI) involve baseline renal function, contrast load, and measures of clinical course [22]. The most widely used and validated score was published by Mehran et al. [23] and utilizes baseline renal function (Cr or Cr clearence), age, gender, hemoglobin, diabetes, history of heart failure, the development of shock requiring intra-aortic balloon counterpulsation. And the volume of contrast adminstered. This score can be calculated after a percutaneous cornary intervention and predicts the risk of CI-AKI and the need for RRT. In the validation subset of the study, there was only fair discrimination for those predicted to develop CI-AKI. (C static = 0.67)

Kidney damage markers have been measured at baseline and serially after exposure (2, 4, 8, 24, and 48h) to iodinated contrast and early injury could be demostrated for both palma and urinary NGAL and L-FABP prior to incease in Scr in several smaller studies in patients with normal renal function at baseline [82, 83]. Urinary IL-18 has also been show to rise in concert with NGAL after contrast exposure [84]. In general, the elevations in novel markers after contrast exposure are less than those after cardiac surgery.

## Nephrotoxin Exposure

A host of important therapeutic agents, such as aminoglycosides and cisplatin, can have direct nephrotoxicity [85, 86]. The ability to predict nephrotoxicity to stop a particular angent in order to reduce risk for AKI and improve patient safety is clinically relevant. There are know risk factors for aminoglycoside nephrotoxicity such as age, diabetes, baseline renal function, duration of therapy of and frequency of dosing [88, 89]. However, to our knowledge, no clinical risk score has been developed in this setting.

Animal studies have suggested that urinary excretion of α-glutathione S-transferase (α-GST), μ-GST, clusterin, and renal papillary antigen-1 could be used to monitor for cisplatin, gentamicin, or N-phenylanthranilic acid-associated nephrotoxicity [90]. In another animal study, KIM-1 appear to detect gentamicin, mercury, and chromium associated associated-nephrotoxicity more readily than other markers including blood urea nitrogen (BUN), Scr and NAG [91]. The US Food and Drug Adminstration and European Medicines Agency have qualified a panel of seven urinary kidney damage bio-markers that were shown in rodent studies to outperform Scr for the identification of nephrotoxicity as assessed by kidney histopathology [92] Thus, a negative or normal panel of kidney damage markers could be an advance in patient safety when performed on a regular basis with the use of common nephrotoxic agents (aminoglycosides, vancomycin, cisplatin, etc.). Clinical studies are clearly needed in this area and are being initiated in the USA through collaboration among several large pharmaceutical companies participating in the Predictive Safety Testing Consortium [92]. These studies will evaluate the performance of several injury bio-markers in patients exposed to cisplatin and apulminoglycosides in two different populations.

## Critical Illness

In critical ill patients admitted to intensive care units (ICU), Cortsidis et al. [93] have developed a clinical risk score including only serum albumin, presence or absence of sepsis and urine osmolality. This score outperformed the APACHE III score to predict AKI or mortality, but was not as preditive in critically ill patients in surgical ICUs [94]. Chawla et al. [95] also developed a clinical score to predict AKI in critically ill patients including many clinical variables. The only variables predictive of AKI were serum albumin concentration, increased A-a gradient, and presence of active cancer.

The published studies to date indicate that upon admission to an ICU or an emergency department, levels of multiple novel markers are predictive for the development of AKI, need for RRT, prolonged length of stay, and death [96-99]. We believe that patient who are considered to be high risk for AKI with both risk factors and renal stressors on admission to the ICU (Table 3), particularly those with sepsis, should be considered as candidates for testing with novel AKI bio-markers. In the absence of critical illness, the serial monitoring of novel markers for the early detection of AKI in sepsis is the current objective of several large, onging observational studies.

## Sepsis

Hospitalized patients with multiple organ system dysfunction, infection, systemic inflammation, with or without obvious hemodynamic perturbations have the highest risk for AKI. Most attempts at risk prediction using clinical variables and or novel bio-markerss have chosen in-hospital mortality as the outcome of interest and not AKI per se [100]. In addition, all risk prediction schemes use variables that in general are poxies for the severity of underlying illness and are not specific, independent predictors for AKI separate from mortality.

Because AKI occuring in the ICU is frequently complicated by sepsis [101] and since sepsis and AKI synergistically increase mortality rate [102], identifying sepsis as the cause of AKI is of great potential significance in clinical management. Plasma NGAL has been reported to be higher in septic than in non-septic AKI patients in several [102, 103], but not all [104] studies. Both sepsis and AKI increased urinary cystatin C and their effects appear to be additive [105]. Similarly, evaluation of five urinary bio-markers (NGAL, Il-18, L-FABP, NAG, and albumin) in a mixed ICU revealed that the highest values were all in septic AKI patient, with L-FABP able to discriminate AKI both septic and non-septic patients (Table 4) [95]. These results suggest that higher thresholds of single and multiple bio-markers may differentiate septic from non-septic AKI.

## The Prognosis of AKI

The current annual expense in the USA for the treatment of acute kidney injury (AKI) is estimated at USD 10 billion [106]. Patients who develop AKI have worse outcomes characterized by higher mortality, prolonged duration of hospitalization and increased risk for progression to CKD [107, 108]. Despite advances in modern medicine the outcomes from AKI have remained relatively unchanged over past few decades [109]. The failure to translate successful interventional strategies from animal models to humans has in part been attributed to the lack of appropriately sensitive and specific bio-markers for timely identification of kidney damage. Over the last decade, several new bio-markers for the timely identification of kidney damage have been characterized and are being validated in clinical studies. These damage bio-markers complement existing conventional bio-markers of kidney function (e.g., Serum Cr, serum urea, and urine output) that are currently utilized to diagnose and stage AKI. Both functional and damage bio-markers provide an opportunity to identify patients with AKI who are at risk for less favorable prognosis in terms of worsening damage or further declines in kidney function, likelihood of need for renal replacement therapy (RRT), non-recovery of kidney function, greater resource uilization, and mortality. However, there are currently no evidence-based or consensus-driven recommendations for the pragmatic utilization of these bio-markers for managing patients with AKI such as identifying time points for interventions predicting outcomes. As additional kidney damage-specific bio-markers are indentified, the integration of both functional and novel damage bio-markers will provide novel opportunities to improve the risk stratification of patients at an earlier stage for referal to renal services and avoid unnecessary delays in treatment and patient transfer. Conversely, the ability of bio-markers to determine that recovery is iminent could forestall the inappropriate commencement of RRT and the risks associated with line insertion (infection and bleeding). Alternatively, the biomarker could indicate that recovery is unlikely in the short term and therefore commencement of RRT is in the best interests of the patient before the development of uremic complications and exposure to non-beneficial medical management such as excessive fluid administration of and/or diuretics. Furthermore, the severity of AKI predicts progression to CKD [110] and thus there is a clinical need to identify patients who are at a high risk of developing progressive kidney disease, rather than complete recovery from AKI. bio-markers could help indentify risk for in complete recovery and long-term progression to CKD and allow the earlier introduction of conventional or even novel interventional therapy.

**Table 4. Five urinary bio-markers in AKI complicated by sepsis**

| | Non-sepsis No-AKI(n = 178) | Non-sepsis (n = 95) | Sepsis No-AKI (n = 30) | Sepsis AKI (n = 36) |
|---|---|---|---|---|
| L-FABP, ng/ml | 6.8(1.5-17.3) | 35.9(6.8-156)[b] | 21.5(4.6-46.1) | 64.5(18.8-543.3)[a] |
| NGAL, ng/ml | 11.5(4.7-33.2) | 32.8(13.3-136.9) | 137.8(39.2-323.5) | 271(118.1-1,593.6)[a] |
| IL-18, pg/ml | 45.3(20.0-110.6) | 122.9(34.5-390.2) | 206.2(133.5-802.1) | 405.0(209.6-1,043.9) |
| NAG, U/l | 7.5(3.8-14.7) | 11.9(5.4-22.6)[b] | 22.8(9.3-40.2) | 22.4(11.9-45.8) |
| Albumin, mg/dl | 2.9(1.1-7.1) | 6.2(3.0-26.5)[b] | 7.8(3.5-21.1) | 15.4(7.4-43.7) |

Values are presented as median (interquartile range). [a] $p < 0.05$ vs. Non-sepsis/non-sepsis/non-AKI, non-sepsis/AKI, and sepsis/non-AKI. [b]$p < 0.05$ vs. Non-sepsis/non-AKI. Data from Doi et al. [95]

## Prediction of Clinically Relevant Outcomes

While there is an abundance of pulications on novel kidney injury bio-markers, most of these data have focused on their ability to predict the development of AKI, generally defined by changes in the currently used functional bio-markers of kidney function (Scr and/or urine out). Some data, however, do exist on the ability of selected bio-markers to provide information above and beyond simple prediction of AKI. These data provide additional prognostic information, including the severity and duration of AKI, likelihood of need to initiation RRT, delayed and/or non-recovery of kidney function and mortality In addition, conventional bio-markers of kidney function (i.e., change in Scr, urine output) have been reassessed to determine their predictive capacity in a contemporary format.

Many of these so-called 'prognostic' biomarker studies have been performed in the setting of timed injury models, such as after cardiac surgery where the onset of injury stimulus is known, and in the ICU settings where multiple insults combine to lead to AKI. For example, in the setting of pediatric cardiac surgery, early postoperative elevations in urinary interleukin (IL)-18, and urinary and plasma neutrophil gelatinase-associated lipocalin (NGAL) were all significantly associated with longer lengths of ICU stay after adjustment for other prognostic factors, and quintiles of each biomarker were also associated with duration of mechanical ventilation postoperatively in multivariable analyses [111]. Also in the setting of pediatric cardiac surgery, Bennett et al. [112] reported that elevated urinary NGAL levels occurring as early as 2h after surgery predicted the severity and duration of AKI, prolonged length of stay, RRT requirement, and death. Serial measurement of urinary kidney injury molecule (KIM)-1 and IL-18 starting prior to and following cardiac surgery with cardiopulmonary bypass (CPB) were correlated with both the diagnosis and likelihood of worsening AKI [113]. Other bio-markers that have been shown to be associated with worsening severity of AKI include plasma cystatin C and urinary π-GST. A prospective study of 123 adults undergoing cardiac surgery found urinary π-GST levels at the time of increase in serum Cr predicted worsening AKI and progression to AKIN stage 3 [114].

In settings where the measurement of selected bio-markers are made at the time of hospital or ICU admission, and hence may not be measured in relative proximity to the time of injury, bio-markers still may appear to have some prognostic utility for adverse outcomes. In a study of more than 500 critically ill adult patients, urinary NGAL, cystatin C, and IL-18 measurements at the time of ICU admission predicted not only AKI, but also worsening AKI and need for RRT [115]. Of interest, in this study the association with adverse outcomes such as hospital mortality was stronger than for AKI itself. In another study of 451 critically ill patients, urinary IL-18 measured within 24h of ICU admission was a strong predictor of death and/or receipt of acute RRT within 28 days. Similar to the previous study, urinary IL-18 predicted hospital mortality but not the development of AKI [116]. Urinary NGAL has also been shown to predict a composite outcome that included worsening severity of AKI in hospitalized patients with estabished AKI [117]. Furthermore, semiquantitative urinary sediment scoring has been shown to have some value in the prognostication of AKI in hospitalized patients receiving a nephrology consult [118]. Development and standardization processing and scoring of urinary sediment currently exist. Hall et al. [119] assessed 249 patients, half of which were critically ill, and compared several novel AKI bio-markers with urine sediment examination to predict adverse outcomes. These data were consistent with additional reports suggesting urine sediment may have added diagnostic and prognostic value to novel AKI bio-markers [120].

In additional, the value of urine output as a biomarker in AKI has recently been reappraised, as there has been incomplete understanding and controversy regarding the precise utility of oliguria in the diagnosis and prognosis of AKI. To understand this further, Macedo et al. [121] utilized high-fidelity urimeters to compare various definitions of oliguria in critical ill patients. The observed incidence of AKI increased significantly from 24-52% when adding the urine output criteria, as defined by the AKIN classification system, to the serum Cr-based criteria alone. When the most conservative measure of oliguria was assessed, patients without a chang in Scr had ICU mortality similar to oliguric patients with an increase in Scr (8.8 vs 10.4%). Moreover, oliguria was a more sensitive marker of AKI, and tended to occur earlier than did change in Scr. These data reaffirm the clinical relevance and importance of the urine output criteria to the AKIN classification system for AKI.

In terms of blood bio-markers, in two large general adult ICU populations, elevated plasma NGAL levels at ICU admission showed very good discriminations of patients who subsequently received RRT, with areas under the receiver operator curve (AuROC) of 0.82-0.88, however, showed only fair prediction of mortality (AuROCs 0.63-0.68) [122, 123]. Plasma NGAL levels also correlated with severity and duration of AKI, as well as general severity of illness scores including Acute Physiology and Chronic Health Evaluation II (APACHEII) [124]. Furthermore, in selected ICU patients with severe AKI treated with RRT, plasma NGAL levels at the time of RRT initiation were higher in non-surviors compared to surviors, and were independently associated with 28-day survival [125]. Serum cystatin C has been reported to be an independent predictor of the severity of AKI after cardiac surgery [126], but prediction of RRT use or composite of RRT and death in ICU or nephrology consult populations have been more modest (AuROCs 0.62-0.76)[127-129].

With regard specifically to RRT, early initiation of renal in selected patients with established AKI may have the potential to improve outcomes [130]. If novel bio-markers were able to predict the need for RRT, they could potentially be used to inform the decision to initiate RRT. A recent review, examining NGAL, cystatin C, NAG, KIM-1, and α1-microgloulin, among others, suggested that selected novel bio-markers have the potential to discriminate earlier in those who will develop worsening AKI and need RRT [131]. However, these data require additional verification due to several limitations, including variation across studies on when RRT is initiates, which results in heterogeity of timing of biomarker measurement and associated variablity in the prognostic predictive value of these measurements [131].

At the moment, few studies have addressed the utility of bio-markers for predicting the timing and extent of kidney recovery (if any) after an episode of AKI. The recovery process depends on several factors, including the severity of the initial injury and whether there are ongoing insults. In a substudy of 76 critically ill non-anuric patients from the Acute Renal Failure Trial Network (ATN), Srisawat et al. [132] examined whether serial changes in urine bio-markers identified those RRT-requiring AKI patients who recovered (i.e., Recovered renal function and were alive at 60 days). While a composite of bio-markers alone, including urinary cystatin c, hepatocyte growth factor, and NGAL achieved AuROC etimates of ~0.7-0.8 for predicting in kidney recovery, improvement in discrimination (AuROC > 0.9) was obstained only after integrating clinical paremeters, such Charlson comorbidity index and APACHE II scores, into the clinical prediction model. The authors concluded that a panel of urine bio-markers can improve clinical risk prediction for non-recovery after AKI. This study highlights a few points. First, given the competing risk of renal recovery and death, it comes as no surprise that when 'recovery' requires both, additional clinical parameters would have to be added to the models to improve their precision. Second, serial measurements of at least two urinary bio-markers are needed to improve precision. Third, despite the heterogeneous precipitants for AKI, these urinary bio-markers appear to have broad prognostic utility. While this study had a small sample size and needs further verification, it highlights an important consideration. An ideal biomarker for a particular disease, such as AKI, should incrementally add value in addition to the baseline clinical risk assessment.

Lastly, in a study on acute heart failure (HF), discharge plasma NGAL level was a stronger predictor of 30-day outcome, including re-hospitalization or death, than brain natriuretic peptide (BNP), the guideline-supported standard for risk prediction, even after adjustment for diacharge kidney function [133]. One could speculate that a high NGAL at the time of discharge following treatment for an episode of acute HF might imply a greater need for surveillance and monitoring following hospital discharge.

## Factors Affecting the Operative Characteristics of Bio-Markers for Prognostication of AKI

Data has increasingly accumulated on several kidney injury bio-markers suggesting that their diagnostic and prognotic performance may vary depending on the clinical setting in which they are evaluated [134]. These observed differences in biomarker performance, across demographic features, co-morbidities and clinical settings have created unique challenges for interpretation and generalizability. These finding suggest that we need to clarify if and to what extent these bio-markers show variable patterns of expression (static and dynamic) across standard demographic features such as age and sex, analogous to age- and sex-specific normative data for conventional measures of kidney function (i.e, serum Cr). The hetergeneity of patients populations, covariates used in multivariable modeling, assay differences, and need for cost-benefit analyses all preclude uniform adaptation of bio-markers into routine clinical pratice at the present time.

CKD is a potentically important modifier of the performance of bio-markers for diagnosis/prognosis in AKI [115, 116, 135]. McIlroy et al. [135] found urine NGAL was a better diagnostic predictor of AKI, defined as an >50% or >0.3mg/dl in Scr, following cardiac surgery in those with a baseline eGFR>= 60ml/min/1.73m2. Siew et al. Found modest improvement in the performance of urine IL-18 for predicting AKI within 24h of ICU admission when stratified by eGFR>= 60ml/min/1.73m2 [116]. Endre et al. [115] also recently reported variable performance of several bio-markers for AKI diagnosis and prediction of outcomes when stratified by both eGFR and by time after kidney insult in a prospective cohort of 529 critically ill patients. At the present time however, there are no such established differentially cut-off values for renal bio-markers among patients with and without CKD.

Other than CKD, there remains uncertainty whether the variable expression of these bio-markers across clinical settings represents differences attributabld to isolate 'kidney injury' or response to increased 'systemic' illness. Experimental models of ischemia-reperfusion injury have clearly improved our understanding of the specific kidney expression of bio-markers such as NGAL [136], however there is uncertainty of how its performance will extended to more general clinical settings. This may account for the inconsistent performance between bio-markers evaluated in relatively isolated settings of AKI, such as cardiac surgery-associated AKI (post-CPB), contrast nephrology, or delayed graft function after kidney transplation, versus more complex multisystem illness settings in which numerous additional confounders may be present (i.e., Sepsis, maligancy) [134]. This would imply there is need for added understanding of not only 'context-specific' performance, but also their time-specific (temporal patterns), and illness severity-specific (non-kidney organ injury) performance. While these bio-markers clearly show correlation with AKI, in particular in models of ischemia-reperfusion and nephrotoxity, selected bio-markers including NGAL [137, 138], IL-18[139], L-FABP[140], can show increased expression with systemic illness and non-kidney organ injurys stimulus can induce secondary organ dysfunction (i.e., kidney-organ crosstalk), and many further bias its opertative performance. For example, increased bio-markers expression in septic AKI compared with non-specific AKI patients has been shown in some studies [141, 142], however not in others [122]. In other words, the high NPV and high PPV cut-off points may be shifted to the right in sepsis. It is unknown how the phase of sepsis (i.e., acute, subacute, recovering) might impact this phenomenon. Moreover, selected data further the diagnostic and prognostic preformance may improve if septic patients are excluded [141, 143].

In summary, it is important that clinicians who intend to use bio-markers in clinical practice be aware that selected bio-markers show variable operative characteristics when stratified by CKD and sepsis. Additional research on selected functional and damage bio-markers is needed for independent validation of across demographic features, selected comorbidities (in particular CKD), and across clinical settings (in particular sepsis) and illness severity.

## Serial Biomarker Measurements for Prognostication in AKI

There remains uncertainty on whether serial biomarker evaluation in patients at-risk for or early after developing AKI can provide additional information for clarifying prognosis.

There have been numerous studies that have described the temporal patterns of biomarker detection in AKI, including after cardiac surgery [111, 112, 113, 144-148] and in critically ill or septic patient [149]. However, few studies have provided any detailed description of the potential added prognostic value of evaluting the rate of or time-average change, the absolute or relative magnitude of change (i.e., delta), or the trajectory of change (i.e., Increasing, decreasing, stable) of selected damage bio-markers after the occurrence of a kidney insult, compared with serial conventional measure of kidney function such as serum Cr. Changes in urine output and patterns of change in serum Cr have been shown to have prognostic information representing alterations in functional bio-markers [121, 150], however these changes have not been correlated with concurrent alterations in damage markers. Moreover, no study has evaluated the potentia additive value of serial biomarker evaluation in reseponse to therapeutic interventions such as acute resusciation, hemodynamic optimization, antimicrobial therapy in sepsis, withdrawl of nephrotoxins, and other novel interventions in the setting of a randomized trial. Such data would be important in determining whether such bio-markers can be used for 'biomonitoring'. In a prospective study of 632 consecutive critically ill patients, de Geus et al. [123] evaluted the diagnostic and prognostic performance of serial plasma and urine NGAL measures early after ICU admission. In this secondary analysis, temporal changes in plasma or urine NGAL during the first 24h did not significantly improve the prediction of development of RIFLE-E, rather the most proximate measure of NGAL temporally associated with achieving RIFLE-F was more predictive.

Serial biomarker evaluation has also been studied for clinical prediction of recovery of kidney function following an episode of AKI. In the above-mentioned substudy of the ATN trial, the addition of the largest relative changes across a panel of urine bio-markers at 14 days, when combined with the most robust clinical risk prediction model, significantly improved overall model performance for predicting kidney recovery [131].

In theory, the use of serial measures of selective bio-markers may have added clinical importance in settings where the time of kidney insult is uncertain and/or where there are multiple temporally separated contributing risks for AKI [115, 151]. The timing of biomarker measurement relative to kidney insult appear to significantly impact its performance for the prediction and/or diagnosis of AKI [115]. Likewise, we need improved understanding of the variability in pathophysiologic expression of kidney injury-specific bio-markers relative to the kidney insult for detecting discrete 'phases' of injury that correlate not only with severity and duration of injury, but also with loss of function and/or clinically important endpoints. It has been postulated that differences in performance for detection of early, sustained or resolving kidney damage may relate to whether the bio-markers is performed and constitutive (i.e., Tubular brush border enzymes) or inducible and upregulated (i.e., NGAL, KIM-1) in the presence of tubular injury. Furthermore, serial biomarker measurements could potentially identify the occurrence of new insult, however studied which address this issue directly are currently lacking.

Clearingly, serial biomarker measurements could potentially add to healthcare costs. In addition to the knowledge gaps already described above, there are no data specifically evaluating the cost-to-benefit ratio of serial measurement in the prognostication of AKI. Overall, while we believe temporal assessment of bio-markers is likely to have value for clarifying prognostic uncertainty, we are unable to recommend a specific serial testing schedule based on the available literature. Further studies are needed to clarify the role of serial measures of selected bio-markers for the diagnosis and projected severity of AKI, clarifying prognostic uncertainty, and for the assessment of kidney-specific response to interventions.

## Bio-Markers and Clinical Management Decisions

Until recently, most clinicians were satisfied with the definition of an ideal biomarker as a sensitive and specific tool for diagnosis of a disease state as well as prognostic for near-term clinical outcomes [152]. More recently, a new updated definition of the ideal biomarker has been proposed [153]. In this paradigm, a 'prognostic' biomarker is only important as a risk-stratifying tool if it is 'clinically actionable' (i.e., it can be used to start a clinically relevant therapy and/or can be used to 'biomonitor' the treatment success or failure).

The early identification of AKI by bio-markers may be particularly 'actionable' in the emergency room (ER) setting, where the potential adverse consequences of sending home a patient with evoloving AKI could be severe. A reduction in urine flow has been demonstrated to be an early phsiologic marker of renal functional change associated with adverse outcomes, particularly when measured accurately [121]. In both adult and ER pediatric settings, NGAL has been shown to identify patients with AKI and who proceed to require higher intensity monitoring and support, such as ICU admission, nephrology consultation and initiation of RRT [154, 155]. In this cotext, it can be useful for clinical triage of patients to either hospital admission. Or at the very least, further evaluation in the ER, perhaps by a nephrologist. In an analogous manner, this could potentially be applied to the ward setting, in that patients with positive bio-markers can be moved to a higher acuity unit with enhanced monitoring capacity. Although this approach has not been tested in a randomized controlled manner, it has potential benefits with (debatably) relatively little foreseeable clinical 'downside'. However, it is acknowledged that monitoring a large number of patients, some of whom will be 'false posivetives', would impact on healthcare costs. This aspect deserves further study.

At least two studies have shown that delayed nephrology consultation can be associated with increased ICU mortality [156, 157]. Lower serum Cr level and higher urine output were associated with delayed consultation, suggesing that these traditional bio-markers may have led to understimation of the severity of kidney dysfunction in these patients. In a separate prospective controlled non-randomized intervention study, a compulsory one-time nephrology consult was performed within 18h of fulfilling AKIN criteria (incease in Scr $\geqq$ 0.3mg/dl) for AKI[158]. In this single-center study, this prompt nephrology consultation was associated with a lower peak serum Cr. The primary outcome of a 2.5 fold increase in serum Cr occured in 12.9% of patients in the control group compared with 3.3% of patients who received early nephrology consultation. In another article in this volume it has been proposed that novel bio-markers be integrated with RIFLE/AKIN for the diagnosis of AKI, specifically that abnormal levels of bio-markers may be used to diagnose AKI even in the absence of changes in serum Cr or oliguria. Patients with elevated bio-markers without diagnostic changes in serum Cr are at higher risk for adverse outcomes, including need for RRT and mortality [159]. Although not yet supported by RCT evidence, we suggested that consultation with clinicians with AKI expertise should be considered in response to elevation in funcional and/or damage bio-markers.

In the absence of specific therapeutic interventions, it may seem curious that the early introduction of nephrology expertise seems to improve outcomes. We believe that this is likely due earlier identification of the important of AKI, consideration for its etiology, and withdrawal or appropriate dose adjustment of potential nephrotoxins, many of which have only been recently identified. In the above-mentioned study [158], the observed effect on peak serum Cr was achieved with fairly simple diagnostic and therapeutic recommendations (Table 5). In another article in this volume it has been recommended that the etiology of AKI should be determined as soon as the diagnosis is made volume. Context-specific bio-markers (i.e, natriuretic peptides, procalcitonin, renal imaging) may assist in determing the etiology and severity of AKI, and could be performed in response to abnormal biomarker levels. Furthermore, renal protective stragies, as listed in Table 5, can be easily implemented. Although the beneficial effect of these interventions was shown in a study in which the trigger was a change in serum Cr, we suggest that these actions can be undertaken at the time of AKI diagnosis, be it by serum Cr, urine output or biomarker.

**Table 5. Potential clinical actions in response to altered biomarker levels**

| **Triage decisions** |
|---|
| *Examples: admitted from ER, hold for further observation, move from award to higher acuity unit* |
| Nephrology consultation |
| Differential diagnosis |
| Search for reversible hemodynamic causes |
| Search for potential direct nephrotoxins |
| Context-specific bio-markers[1], imaging and other studies to establish AKI etiology |
| Renoprotective strategies |
| Higher acuity monitoring(fluid balance, urine output, creatinine, blood pressure, cardiac function) |
| Hold ACE-I/ARB |
| Optimize volume status and perfusion pressure |
| Adjust diuretic doses |
| Initial use of vasodilators, including nitrates, hydralazine and nesiritide (in acute heart failure) |
| Pharmacovigilance (drug monitoring/dosing, avoiding nephrotoxins, attention to drug interactions) |
| Radiocontrast precautions/consider alternative to radiocontrast procedures |
| Supportive management |
| Avoid hyperglycemia |
| Anticipate AKI complications (e.g., Hyperkalemia, volume overload, etc.) |
| Consider adjusting nutrition (e.g., Attention to K, PO4 content, volume, etc.) |
| Consider timely initiation of renal support |
| Avoid subclavian catheters if possible |
| Context-specific intervention(s) |
| Consider early or close follow up |

[1]example of context-specific bio-markers: BNP and NT-proBNP for heart failure; bilirubin and hepatic enzymes for hepatic failure; procalcitonin, endotoxin activity assay an culture for sepsis.

Based on the clinical context, there are data to suggest selected bio-markers can be important tools to aid in patient triage and management decisions (e.g., Renal protective strategies, nephrology consultation). Biomarker assays have been introduced in some countries but their clinical uptake has not been high enough to develop a knowledge base of thresholds, however based on published observational studies of these bio-markers, potential thresholds can be suggested but will need to be validated. Additional research must clarify the optimal biomarker values for categorizing high PPV/NPV for specific clinical management decisions. Furthermore, research on cost-benefit assessment of such biomarker guided clinical action plans is needed.

## CONCLUSION

Understanding of baseline risk factors, renal stressor, and incorporation of the results of novel kidney damage markers (either assessed in blood or urine, or via other innovative physiological or imaging measures) may provide a step forward in avoiding harm to the kidney and improving patient safety and devise early the preventive strategies. Several novel kidney damage bio-markers are now commercially available for AKI diagnosis, including blood and urine NGAL and L-FABP. We recognize that other markers are in late-stage clinical development and may in fact be superior to the ones currently available. We recommend that novel kidney damage bio-markers be integrated with the RIFLE/AKIN criteria for diagnosis of AKI. In the appropriate clinical setting, AKI may be diagnosed by either an abnormal damage biomarker or change in Scr or UO. This new damage criterion will complement the ability of RIFLE/AKIN to define AKI. There are insufficient data on damage bio-markers to support their use for staging of AKI. At initial evaluation, patients can categorized into one of the four diagnostic categories that each would have potential clinical significance with respect to outcome. Carefully constructed clinical research to guide this field will be critical to determine whether the additional cost is worthwhile and to leverage outcomes for benefit in this population.

## References


[1] KDIGO, AKI. Guidelines: Summary of recommendation statements. *Kidney Int Suppl*, 2012, 2, 8-12.

[2] Uchino, S; Bellomo, R; Goldsmith, D; Bate, S; Ronco, C. An assessment of the RIFLE criteria for acute renal failure in hospitalized patients. *Crit Care Med*, 2006, 34, 1913-1917.

[3] Waikar, SS; Bonventre, JV. Cr kinetics and the definition of acute kidney injury. *J Am Soc Nephrol*, 2009, 20, 672-679.

[4] Himmelfarb, J; Ikizler, TA. Acute kidney injury: changing lexicography, definitions, and epidemiology. *Kidney Int.*, 2007 May, 71(10), 971-976.

[5] Prowle, JR; Liu, YL; Licari, E; Bagshaw, SM; Egi, M; Haase, M; Haase-Fielitz, A; Kellum, JA; Cruz, D; Ronco, C; Tsutsui, K; Uchino, S; Bellomo, R. Oliguria as predictive biomarker of acute kidney injury in critically ill patients. *Crit Care.*, 2011 Jul 19, 15(4), R172.

[6] Haase, M; Devarajan, P; Haase-Fielitz, A; Bellomo, R; Cruz, DN; Wagener, G; Krawczeski, CD; Koyner, JL; Murray, P; Zappitelli, M; Goldstein, SL; Makris, K; Ronco, C; Martensson, J; Martling, CR; Venge, P; Siew, E; Ware, LB; Ikizler, TA; Mertens, PR. The outcome of neutrophil gelatinase-associated lipocalin-positive subclinical acute kidney injury: a multicenter pooled analysis of prospective studies. *J Am Coll Cardiol*, 2011, 57, 1752-1761.

[7] Boudonck, KJ; Rose, DJ; Karoly, ED; Lee, DP; Lawton, KA; Lapinskas, PJ. Metabolomics for early detection of drug-induced kidney injury: review of the current status. *Bioanalysis*, 2009, 1, 1645-1663.

[8] McCullough, PA; Chinnaiyan, KM; Gallagher, MJ; Colar, JM; Geddes, T; Gold, JM; Trivax, JE. Changes in renal markers and acute kidney injury after marathon running. *Nephrology* (Carlton)., 2011, 16, 194-199.

[9] Kashani, K; Al-Khafaji, A; Ardiles, T; Artigas, A; et al. Discovery and validation of cell cycle arrest bio-markers in human acute kidney injury. *Critcal Care*, 2013, 17, R25.

[10] Doi, K; Negishi, K; Ishizu, T; Katagiri, D; Fujita, T; Matsubara, T; Yahagi, N; Sugaya, T; Noiri, E. Evaluation of new acute kidney injury bio-markers in a mixed intensive care unit. *Critcal Care*, 2011, 39, 2464-2469.

[11] Prowle, JR; Liu, YL; Licari, E; Bagshaw, SM; Egi, M; Haase, M; Haase-Fielitz, A; Kellum, JA; Cruz, D; Ronco, C; Tsutsui, K; Uchino, S;

Bellomo, R. Oliguria as predictive biomarker of acute kidney injury in critically ill patients. *Criti Care*, 2011, 15, R172.

[12] Sutton, TA; Fisher, CJ; Molitoris BA. Microvascular endothelial injury and dysfunction during ischemic acute renal failure. *Kidney Int*, 2002, 62, 1539-1549.

[13] Welch, WJ. Intrarenal oxygen and hypertension. *Clin Exp Pharmacol Physiol.*, 2006 Oct, 33(10), 1002-5.

[14] Evans, RG; Gardiner, BS; Smith, DW; O'Connor, PM. Intrarenal oxygenation: unique challenges and the biophysical basis of homeostasis. *Am J Physiol Renal Physiol.*, 2008 Nov, 295(5), F1259-70.

[15] Hostetter, TH. Human renal response to meat meal. *Am J Physiol.*, 1986 Apr, 250(4 Pt 2), F613-8.

[16] Legrand, M; Mik, EG; Balestra, GM; Lutter, R; Pirracchio, R; Payen, D. Ince CFluid resuscitation does not improve renal oxygenation during hemorrhagic shock in rats. *Anesthesiology*, 2010, 112, 119-127.

[17] Le Dorze, M; Legrand, M; Payen, D; Ince, C. The role of the microcirculation in acute kidney injury. *Curr Opin Crit Care*, 2009, 15, 503-508.

[18] Kalantarinia, K; Belcik, JT; Patrie, JT; Wei, K. Real-time measurement of renal blood flow in healthy subjects using contrast-enhanced ultrasound. *Am J Physiol Renal Physiol.*, 2009 Oct, 297(4), F1129-34.

[19] Dagher, PC; Herget-Rosenthal, S; Ruehm, SG; Jo, SK; Star, RA; Agarwal, R; Molitoris, BA. Newly developed techniques to study and diagnose acute renal failure. *J Am Soc Nephrol.* 2003 Aug, 14(8), 2188-98.

[20] Schock-Kusch, D; Xie, Q; Shulhevich, Y; Hesser, J; Stsepankou, D; Sadick, M; Koenig, S; Hoecklin, F; Pill, J; Gretz, N. Transcutaneous assessment of renal function in conscious rats with a device for measuring FITC-sinistrin disappearance curves. *Kidney Int.*, 2011 Jun, 79(11), 1254-8.

[21] Wang, E; Meier, DJ; Sandoval, RM; Von Hendy-Willson, VE; Pressler, BM; Bunch, RM; Alloosh, M; Sturek, MS; Schwartz, GJ; Molitoris, BA. A portable fiberoptic ratiometric fluorescence analyzer provides rapid point-of-care determination of glomerular filtration rate in large animals. *Kidney Int.*, 2012 Jan, 81(1), 112-7.

[22] Bellomo, R; Ronco, C; Kellum, JA; Mehta, RL; Palevsky, P. Acute Dialysis Quality Initiative workgroup. Acute renal failure – definition, outcome measures, animal models, fluid therapy and information technology needs: the Second International Consensus Conference of the

Acute Dialysis Quality Initiative (ADQI) Group. *Crit Care.*, 2004 Aug, 8(4), R204-12.

[23] Mehta, RL; Kellum, JA; Shah, SV; Molitoris, BA; Ronco, C; Warnock, DG; Levin, A. Acute Kidney Injury Network. Acute Kidney Injury Network: report of an initiative to improve outcomes in acute kidney injury. *Crit Care.*, 2007, 11(2), R31.

[24] Macedo, E; Bouchard, J; Soroko, SH; Chertow, GM; Himmelfarb, J; Ikizler, TA; Paganini, EP; Mehta, RL. Fluid accumulation; recognition and staging of acute kidney injury in critically-ill patients. *Crit Care.*, 2010, 14(3), R82.

[25] Stevens, LA; Coresh, J; Greene, T; Levey, AS. Assessing kidney function--measured and estimated glomerular filtration rate. *N Engl J Med.*, 2006 Jun 8, 354(23), 2473-83.

[26] Macedo, E; Malhotra, R; Claure-Del Granado, R; Fedullo, P; Mehta, RL. Defining urine output criterion for acute kidney injury in critically ill patients. *Nephrol Dial Transplant*, 2011, 26, 509-515.

[27] Hersch, M; Einav, S; Izbicki, G. Accuracy and ease of use of a novel electronic urine output monitoring device compared with standard manual urinometer in the intensive care unit. *J Crit Care.*, 2009 Dec, 24(4), 629. e13-7.

[28] Espinel, CH; Gregory, AW. Differential diagnosis of acute renal failure. *Clin Nephrol*, 1980, 13, 73-77.

[29] Zarich, S; Fang, LS; Diamond, JR. Fractional excretion of sodium. Exceptions to its diagnostic value. *Arch Intern Med.*, 1985 Jan, 145(1), 108-12.

[30] Pépin, MN; Bouchard, J; Legault, L; Ethier, J. Diagnostic performance of fractional excretion of urea and fractional excretion of sodium in the evaluations of patients with acute kidney injury with or without diuretic treatment. *Am J Kidney Dis.*, 2007 Oct, 50(4), 566-73.

[31] Keogan, MT; Kliewer, MA; Hertzberg, BS; DeLong, DM; Tupler, RH; Carroll, BA. Renal resistive indexes: variability in Doppler US measurement in a healthy population. *Radiology.*, 1996 Apr, 199(1), 165-9.

[32] Splendiani, G; Parolini, C; Fortunato, L; Sturniolo, A; Costanzi, S. Resistive index in chronic nephropathies: predictive value of renal outcome. *Clin Nephrol*, 2002, 57, 45-50.

[33] Sugiura, T; Nakamori, A; Wada, A; Fukuhara, Y. Evaluation of tubulointerstitial injury by Doppler ultrasonography in glomerular diseases. *Clin Nephrol.*, 2004 Feb, 61(2), 119-26.

[34] Derchi, LE; Leoncini, G; Parodi, D; Viazzi, F; Martinoli, C; Ratto, E; Vettoretti, S; Vaccaro, V; Falqui, V; Tomolillo, C; Deferrari, G; Pontremoli, R. Mild renal dysfunction and renal vascular resistance in primary hypertension. *Am J Hypertens*, 2005, 18, 966-971.

[35] Akgul, A; Ibis, A; Sezer, S; Basaran, C; Usluogullari, A; Ozdemir, FN; Arat, Z; Haberal, M. Early assessment of renal resistance index and long-term renal function in renal transplant recipients. *Ren Fail*, 2009, 31, 18-24.

[36] Platt, JF; Rubin, JM; Ellis, JH. Acute renal obstruction: evaluation with intrarenal duplex Doppler and conventional US. *Radiology.*, 1993 Mar, 186(3), 685-8.

[37] Lerolle, N; Guérot, E; Faisy, C; Bornstain, C; Diehl, JL; Fagon, JY. Renal failure in septic shock: predictive value of Doppler-based renal arterial resistive index. *Intensive Care Med*, 2006, 32, 1553-1559.

[38] Darmon, M; Schortgen, F; Vargas, F; Liazydi, A; Schlemmer, B; Brun-Buisson, C; Brochard, L. Diagnostic accuracy of Doppler renal resistive index for reversibility of acute kidney injury in critically ill patients. *Intensive Care Med*, 2011, 37, 68-76.

[39] Platt, JF; Rubin, JM; Ellis, JH. Acute renal failure: possible role of duplex Doppler US in distinction between acute prerenal failure and acute tubular necrosis. Radiology., 1991 May, 179(2), 419-23.

[40] Deruddre, S; Cheisson, G; Mazoit, JX; Vicaut, E; Benhamou, D; Duranteau, J. Renal arterial resistance in septic shock: effects of increasing mean arterial pressure with norepinephrine on the renal resistive index assessed with Doppler ultrasonography. *Intensive Care Med*, 2007, 33, 1557-1562.

[41] Klibanov, AL. Ultrasound contrast agents: development of the field and current status. *Top Curr Chem*, 2002, 222, 73-106.

[42] Kishimoto, N; Mori, Y; Nishiue, T; Nose, A; Kijima, Y; Tokoro, T; Yamahara, H; Okigaki, M; Kosaki, A; Iwasaka, T. Ultrasound evaluation of valsartan therapy for renal cortical perfusion. *Hypertens Res*, 2004, 27, 345-349.

[43] Ciccone, MM; Cortese, F; Fiorella, A; Scicchitano, P; Cito, F; Quistelli, G; Pertosa, G; D'Agostino, R; Guida, P; Favale, S. The clinical role of contrast-enhanced ultrasound in the evaluation of renal artery stenosis and diagnostic superiority as compared to traditional echo-color-Doppler flow imaging. *Int Angiol*, 2011, 30, 135-139.

[44] Benozzi, L; Cappelli, G; Granito, M; Davoli, D; Favali, D; Montecchi, MG; Grossi, A; Torricelli, P; Albertazzi, A. Contrast-enhanced

sonography in early kidney graft dysfunction. *Transplant Proc*, 2009, 41, 1214-1215.

[45] Schwenger, V; Korosoglou, G; Hinkel, UP; Morath, C; Hansen, A; Sommerer, C; Dikow, R; Hardt, S; Schmidt, J; Kücherer, H; Katus, HA; Zeier, M. Real-time contrast-enhanced sonography of renal transplant recipients predicts chronic allograft nephropathy. *Am J Transplant*, 2006, 6, 609-615.

[46] Di Iorio, BR; Scalfi, L; Terracciano, V; Bellizzi, V. A systematic evaluation of bioelectrical impedance measurement after hemodialysis session. *Kidney Int*, 2004, 65, 2435-2440.

[47] Juillard, L; Janier, MF; Fouque, D; Lionnet, M; Le Bars, D; Cinotti, L; Barthez, P; Gharib, C; Laville, M. Renal blood flow measurement by positron emission tomography using 15O-labeled water. *Kidney Int*, 2000, 57, 2511-2518.

[48] Alpert, NM; Rabito, CA; Correia, DJ; Babich, JW; Littman, BH; Tompkins, RG; Rubin, NT; Rubin, RH; Fischman, AJ. Mapping of local renal blood flow with PET and H(2)(15)O. *J Nucl Med.*, 2002 Apr, 43(4), 470-5.

[49] Reuter, S; Schnöckel, U; Schröter, R; Schober, O; Pavenstädt, H; Schäfers, M; Gabriëls, Schlatter. Non-invasive imaging of acute renal allograft rejection in rats using small animal F-FDG-PET. *PLoS One.*, 2009, 4(4), e5296.

[50] Petrova, A; Mehta, R. Near-infrared spectroscopy in the detection of regional tissue oxygenation during hypoxic events in preterm infants undergoing critical care. *Pediatr Crit Care Med*, 2006, 7, 449-454.

[51] Ortmann, LA; Fontenot, EE; Seib, PM; Eble, BK; Brown, R; Bhutta, AT. Use of near-infrared spectroscopy for estimation of renal oxygenation in children with heart disease. *Pediatr Cardiol.*, 2011 Aug, 32(6), 748-53.

[52] Dani, C; Pratesi, S; Fontanelli, G; Barp, J; Bertini, G. Blood transfusions increase cerebral, splanchnic, and renal oxygenation in anemic preterm infants. *Transfusion*, 2010, 50, 1220-1226.

[53] Owens, GE; King, K; Gurney, JG; Charpie, JR. Low renal oximetry correlates with acute kidney injury after infant cardiac surgery. *Pediatr Cardiol*, 2011, 32, 183-188.

[54] Yamamoto, T; Hayashi, K; Matsuda, H; Tomura, Y; Ogasawara, Y; Hashimoto, R; Tada, T; Tanaka, H; Kajiya, F. Direct *in vivo* visualization of glomerular microcirculation by intravital pencil lens-

probe CCD videomicroscopy. *Clin Hemorheol Microcirc*, 2000, 23, 103-108.

[55] Scheeren, TW; Martin, K; Maruschke, M; Hakenberg, OW. Prognostic value of intraoperative renal tissue oxygenation measurement on early renal transplant function. *Transpl Int*, 2011, 24, 687-696.

[56] Prasad, PV; Chen, Q; Goldfarb, JW; Epstein, FH; Edelman, RR. Breath-hold R2* mapping with a multiple gradient-recalled echo sequence: application to the evaluation of intrarenal oxygenation. *J Magn Reson Imaging.*, 1997 Nov-Dec, 7(6), 1163-5.

[57] Djamali, A; Sadowski, EA; Muehrer, RJ; Reese, S; Smavatkul, C; Vidyasagar, A; Fain, SB; Lipscomb, RC; Hullett, DH; Samaniego-Picota, M; Grist, TM; Becker, BN. BOLD-MRI assessment of intrarenal oxygenation and oxidative stress in patients with chronic kidney allograft dysfunction. *Am J Physiol Renal Physiol*, 2007, 292, F513-F522.

[58] Wang, ZJ; Kumar, R; Banerjee, S; Hsu, CY. Blood oxygen level-dependent (BOLD) MRI of diabetic nephropathy: preliminary experience. *J Magn Reson Imaging.*, 2011 Mar, 33(3), 655-60.

[59] Thoeny, HC; Zumstein, D; Simon-Zoula, S; Eisenberger, U; De Keyzer, F; Hofmann, L; Vock, P; Boesch, C; Frey, FJ; Vermathen, P. Functional evaluation of transplanted kidneys with diffusion-weighted and BOLD MR imaging: initial experience. *Radiology.*, 2006 Dec, 241(3), 812-21.

[60] Textor, SC; Glockner, JF; Lerman, LO; Misra, S; McKusick, MA; Riederer, SJ; Grande, JP; Gomez, SI; Romero, JC. The use of magnetic resonance to evaluate tissue oxygenation in renal artery stenosis. *J Am Soc Nephrol.*, 2008 Apr, 19(4), 780-8.

[61] Pedersen, M; Dissing, TH; Mørkenborg, J; Stødkilde-Jørgensen, H; Hansen, LH; Pedersen, LB; Grenier, N; Frøkiaer, J. Validation of quantitative BOLD MRI measurements in kidney: application to unilateral ureteral obstruction. *Kidney Int*, 2005, 67, 2305-2312.

[62] Juillard, L; Lerman, LO; Kruger, DG; Haas, JA; Rucker, BC; Polzin, JA; Riederer, SJ; Romero, JC. Blood oxygen level-dependent measurement of acute intra-renal ischemia. *Kidney Int*, 2004, 65, 944-950.

[63] Han, F; Xiao, W; Xu, Y; Wu, J; Wang, Q; Wang, H; Zhang, M; Chen, J. The significance of BOLD MRI in differentiation between renal transplant rejection and acute tubular necrosis. *Nephrol Dial Transplant*, 2008, 23, 2666-2672.

[64] Shaw, AD; Li, Z; Thomas, Z; Stevens, CW. Assessment of tissue oxygen tension: comparison of dynamic fluorescence quenching and polarographic electrode technique. *Crit Care*, 2002, 6, 76-80.

[65] Wang, ZJ; Joe, BN; Coakley, FV; Zaharchuk, G; Busse, R; Yeh, BM. Urinary oxygen tension measurement in humans using magnetic resonance imaging. *Acad Radiol*, 2008, 15, 1467-1473.

[66] LEONHARDT, KO; LANDES, RR. Oxygen tension of the urine and renal structures. Preliminary report of clinical findings. *N Engl J Med.*, 1963 Jul 18, 269, 115-21.

[67] Morelli, A; Rocco, M; Conti, G; Orecchioni, A; Alberto De Blasi, R; Coluzzi, F; Pietropaoli, P. Monitoring renal oxygen supply in critically-ill patients using urinary oxygen tension. *Anesth Analg*, 2003, 97, 1764-1768.

[68] Kainuma, M; Yamada, M; Miyake, T. Continuous urine oxygen tension monitoring in patients undergoing cardiac surgery. *J Cardiothorac Vasc Anesth.*, 1996 Aug, 10(5), 603-8.

[69] Stafford-Smith, M; Podgoreanu, M; Swaminathan, M; Phillips-Bute, B; Mathew, JP; Hauser, EH; Winn, MP; Milano, C; Nielsen, DM; Smith, M; Morris, R; Newman, MF; Schwinn, DA. Perioperative Genetics and Safety Outcomes Study (PEGASUS) Investigative Team. Association of genetic polymorphisms with risk of renal injury after coronary bypass graft surgery. *Am J Kidney Dis.*, 2005 Mar, 45(3), 519-30.

[70] Du Cheyron, D; Fradin, S; Ramakers, M; Terzi, N; Guillotin, D; Bouchet, B; Daubin, C; Charbonneau, P. Angiotensin converting enzyme insertion/deletion genetic polymorphism: its impact on renal function in critically ill patients. *Crit Care Med*, 2008, 36, 3178-3183.

[71] Haase-Fielitz, A; Haase, M; Bellomo, R; Lambert, G; Matalanis, G; Story, D; Doolan, L; Buxton, B; Gutteridge, G; Luft, FC; Schunck, WH; Dragun, D. Decreased catecholamine degradation associates with shock and kidney injury after cardiac surgery. *J Am Soc Nephrol*, 2009, 20, 1393-1403.

[72] Vehaskari, VM. Prenatal programming of kidney disease. *Curr Opin Pediatr*, 2010, 22, 176-182.

[73] McCullough, PA; Lepor, NE. The deadly triangle of anemia, renal insufficiency, and cardiovascular disease: implications for prognosis and treatment. *Rev Cardiovasc Med*, 2005, 6, 1-10.

[74] Goldstein, SL; Chawla, LS. Renal angina. *clin J Am Soc Nephrol*, 2010, 5, 943-949.

[75] Vives, M; Monedero, P; Perez-Valdivieso, JR; Garcia-Fernandez, N; Lavilla, J; Herreros, J; Bes-Rastrollo, M. Spanish Renal Dysfunction in Cardiac Surgery Group. External validation and comparison of three scores to predict renal replacement therapy after cardiac surgery: a multicenter cohort. *Int J Artif Organs*, 2011, 34, 329-338.

[76] Heise, D; Sundermann, D; Braeuer, A; Quintel, M. Validation of a clinical score to determine the risk of acute renal failure after cardiac surgery. *Eur J Cardiothorac Surg*, 2010, 37, 710-716.

[77] Englberger, L; Suri, RM; Li, Z; Dearani, JA; Park, SJ; Sundt, TM; 3rd, Schaff, HV. Validation of clinical scores predicting severe acute kidney injury after cardiac surgery. *Am J Kidney Dis*, 2010, 56, 623-631.

[78] Mehta, RH; Honeycutt, E; Patel, UD; Lopes, RD; Williams, JB; Shaw, LK; O'Brien, SM; Califf, RM; Hughes, GC; Sketch, MH. Jr. Relationship of the time interval between cardiac catheterization and elective coronary artery bypass surgery with postprocedural acute kidney injury. *Circulation.*, 2011 Sep 13, 124(11 Suppl), S149-55.

[79] Parikh, CR; Coca, SG; Thiessen-Philbrook, H; Shlipak, MG; Koyner, JL; Wang, Z; Edelstein, CL; Devarajan, P; Patel, UD; Zappitelli, M; Krawczeski, CD; Passik, CS; Swaminathan, M; Garg, AX. TRIBE-AKI Consortium. Postoperative bio-markers predict acute kidney injury and poor outcomes after adult cardiac surgery. *J Am Soc Nephrol*, 2011, 22, 1748-1757.

[80] Krawczeski, CD; Goldstein, SL; Woo, JG; Wang, Y; Piyaphanee, N; Ma, Q; Bennett, M; Devarajan, P. Temporal relationship and predictive value of urinary acute kidney injury bio-markers after pediatric cardiopulmonary bypass. *J Am Coll Cardiol*, 2011, 58, 2301-2309.

[81] Parikh, CR; Devarajan, P; Zappitelli, M; Sint, K; Thiessen-Philbrook, H; Li, S; Kim, RW; Koyner, JL; Coca, SG; Edelstein, CL; Shlipak, MG; Garg, AX; Krawczeski, CD. TRIBE-AKI Consortium. Postoperative bio-markers predict acute kidney injury and poor outcomes after pediatric cardiac surgery. *J Am Soc Nephrol*, 2011, 22, 1737-1747.

[82] Bachorzewska-Gajewska, H; Malyszko, J; Sitniewska, E; Malyszko, JS; Dobrzycki, S. Neutrophil-gelatinase-associated lipocalin and renal function after percutaneous coronary interventions. *Am J Nephrol.*, 2006, 26(3), 287-92.

[83] Bachorzewska-Gajewska, H; Malyszko, J; Sitniewska, E; Malyszko, JS; Poniatowski, B; Pawlak, K; Dobrzycki, S. NGAL (neutrophil gelatinase-associated lipocalin) and cystatin C: are they good predictors of contrast nephropathy after percutaneous coronary interventions in patients with

stable angina and normal serum Cr? *Int J Cardiol.*, 2008 Jul 4, 127(2), 290-1.

[84] Ling, W; Zhaohui, N; Ben, H; Leyi, G; Jianping, L; Huili, D; Jiaqi, Q. Urinary IL-18 and NGAL as early predictive bio-markers in contrast-induced nephropathy after coronary angiography. *Nephron Clin Pract.*, 2008, 108(3), c176-81.

[85] Perazella, MA; Moeckel, GW. Nephrotoxicity from chemotherapeutic agents: clinical manifestations, pathobiology, and prevention/therapy. *Semin Nephrol*, 2010, 30, 570-581.

[86] Bertino, JS; Jr, Booker, LA; Franck, PA; Jenkins, PL; Franck, KR; Nafziger, AN. Incidence of and significant risk factors for aminoglycoside-associated nephrotoxicity in patients dosed by using individualized pharmacokinetic monitoring. *J Infect Dis.*, 1993 Jan, 167(1), 173-9.

[87] Munckhof, WJ; Grayson, ML; Turnidge, JD. A meta-analysis of studies on the safety and efficacy of aminoglycosides given either once daily or as divided doses. *J Antimicrob Chemother*, 1996, 37, 645-663.

[88] Coritsidis, GN; Guru, K; Ward, L; Bashir, R; Feinfeld, DA; Carvounis, CP. Prediction of acute renal failure by “bedside formula” in medical and surgical intensive care patients. *Ren Fail*, 2000, 22, 235-244.

[89] Munckhof, WJ; Grayson, ML; Turnidge, JD. A meta-analysis of studies on the safety and efficacy of aminoglycosides given either once daily or as divided doses. *J Antimicrob Chemother*, 1996, 37, 645-663.

[90] Harpur, E; Ennulat, D; Hoffman, D; Betton, G; Gautier, JC; Riefke, B; Bounous, D; Schuster, K; Beushausen, S; Guffroy, M; Shaw, M; Lock, E; Pettit, S. HESI Committee on bio-markers of Nephrotoxicity. Biological qualification of bio-markers of chemical-induced renal toxicity in two strains of male rat. *Toxicol Sci.*, 2011 Aug, 122(2), 235-52.

[91] Zhou, Y; Vaidya, VS; Brown, RP; Zhang, J; Rosenzweig, BA; Thompson, KL; Miller, TJ; Bonventre, JV; Goering, PL. Comparison of kidney injury molecule-1 and other nephrotoxicity bio-markers in urine and kidney following acute exposure to gentamicin, mercury, and chromium. *Toxicol Sci*, 2008, 101, 159-170.

[92] Dieterle, F; Sistare, F; Goodsaid, F; Papaluca, M; Ozer, JS; Webb, CP; Baer, W; Senagore, A; Schipper, MJ; Vonderscher, J; Sultana, S; Gerhold, DL; Phillips, JA; Maurer, G; Carl, K; Laurie, D; Harpur, E; Sonee, M; Ennulat, D; Holder, D; Andrews-Cleavenger, D; Gu, YZ; Thompson, KL; Goering, PL; Vidal, JM; Abadie, E; Maciulaitis, R;

Jacobson-Kram, D; Defelice, AF; Hausner, EA; Blank, M; Thompson, A; Harlow, P; Throckmorton, D; Xiao, S; Xu, N; Taylor, W; Vamvakas, S; Flamion, B; Lima, BS; Kasper, P; Pasanen, M; Prasad, K; Troth, S; Bounous, D; Robinson-Gravatt, D; Betton, G; Davis, MA; Akunda, J. Renal biomarker qualification submission: a dialog between the FDA-EMEA and Predictive Safety Testing Consortium. *Nat Biotechnol*, 2010, 28, 455-462.

[93] Coritsidis, GN; Guru, K; Ward, L; Bashir, R; Feinfeld, DA; Carvounis, CP. Prediction of acute renal failure by "bedside formula" in medical and surgical intensive care patients. *Ren Fail*, 2000, 22, 235-244.

[94] Chawla, LS; Abell, L; Mazhari, R; Egan, M; Kadambi, N; Burke, HB; Junker, C; Seneff, MG; Kimmel, PL. Identifying critically ill patients at high risk for developing acute renal failure: a pilot study. *Kidney Int*, 2005, 68, 2274-2280.

[95] Doi, K; Negishi, K; Ishizu, T; Katagiri, D; Fujita, T; Matsubara, T; Yahagi, N; Sugaya, T; Noiri, E. Evaluation of new acute kidney injury bio-markers in a mixed intensive care unit. *Crit Care Med*, 2011, 39, 2464-2469.

[96] de Geus, HR; Bakker, J; Lesaffre, EM; le Noble, JL. Neutrophil gelatinase-associated lipocalin at ICU admission predicts for acute kidney injury in adult patients. *Am J Respir Crit Care Med.*, 2011 Apr 1, 183(7), 907-14.

[97] Shapiro, NI; Trzeciak, S; Hollander, JE; Birkhahn, R; Otero, R; Osborn, TM; Moretti, E; Nguyen, HB; Gunnerson, K; Milzman, D; Gaieski, DF; Goyal, M; Cairns, CB; Kupfer, K; Lee, SW; Rivers, EP. The diagnostic accuracy of plasma neutrophil gelatinase-associated lipocalin in the prediction of acute kidney injury in emergency department patients with suspected sepsis. *Ann Emerg Med*, 2010, 56, 52-59.

[98] Siew, ED; Ware, LB; Gebretsadik, T; Shintani, A; Moons, KG; Wickersham, N; Bossert, F; Ikizler, TA. Urine neutrophil gelatinase-associated lipocalin moderately predicts acute kidney injury in critically ill adults. *J Am Soc Nephrol*, 2009, 20, 1823-1832.

[99] Siew, ED; Ikizler, TA; Gebretsadik, T; Shintani, A; Wickersham, N; Bossert, F; Peterson, JF; Parikh, CR; May, AK; Ware, LB. Elevated urinary IL-18 levels at the time of ICU admission predict adverse clinical outcomes. *Clin J Am Soc Nephrol*, 2010, 5, 1497-1505.

[100] Doi, K; Negishi, K; Ishizu, T; Katagiri, D; Fujita, T; Matsubara, T; Yahagi, N; Sugaya, T; Noiri, E. Evaluation of new acute kidney injury bio-markers in a mixed intensive care unit. *Crit Care Med*, 2011.

[101] Uchino, S; Kellum, JA; Bellomo, R; Doig, GS; Morimatsu, H; Morgera, S; Schetz, M; Tan, I; Bouman, C; Macedo, E; Gibney, N; Tolwani, A; Ronco, C. Beginning and Ending Supportive Therapy for the Kidney (BEST Kidney) Investigators. Acute renal failure in critically ill patients: a multinational, multicenter study. *JAMA.*, 2005 Aug 17, 294(7), 813-8.

[102] Bagshaw, SM; Bennett, M; Haase, M; Haase-Fielitz, A; Egi, M; Morimatsu, H; D'amico, G; Goldsmith, D; Devarajan, P; Bellomo, R. Plasma and urine neutrophil gelatinase-associated lipocalin in septic versus non-septic acute kidney injury in critical illness. *Intensive Care Med.*, 2010 Mar, 36(3), 452-61.

[103] Kümpers, P; Hafer, C; Lukasz, A; Lichtinghagen, R; Brand, K; Fliser, D; Faulhaber-Walter, R; Kielstein, JT. Serum neutrophil gelatinase-associated lipocalin at inception of renal replacement therapy predicts survival in critically ill patients with acute kidney injury. *Crit Care.*, 2010, 14(1), R9.

[104] Mårtensson, J; Bell, M; Oldner, A; Xu, S; Venge, P; Martling, CR. Neutrophil gelatinase-associated lipocalin in adult septic patients with and without acute kidney injury. *Intensive Care Med*, 2010, 36, 1333-1340.

[105] Nejat, M; Pickering, JW; Walker, RJ; Westhuyzen, J; Shaw, GM; Frampton, CM; Endre, ZH. Urinary cystatin C is diagnostic of acute kidney injury and sepsis, and predicts mortality in the intensive care unit. *Crit Care.*, 2010, 14(3), R85.

[106] Fischer, MJ; Brimhall, BB; Lezotte, DC; Glazner, JE; Parikh, CR. Uncomplicated acute renal failure and hospital resource utilization: a retrospective multicenter analysis. *Am J Kidney Dis.*, 2005 Dec, 46(6), 1049-57.

[107] Bagshaw, SM; Laupland, KB; Doig, CJ; Mortis, G; Fick, GH; Mucenski, M; Godinez-Luna, T; Svenson, LW; Rosenal, T. Prognosis for long-term survival and renal recovery in critically ill patients with severe acute renal failure: a population-based study. *Crit Care.*, 2005, 9(6), R700-9.

[108] Ponte, B; Felipe, C; Muriel, A; Tenorio, MT; Liaño, F. Long-term functional evolution after an acute kidney injury: a 10-year study. *Nephrol Dial Transplant*, 2008, 23, 3859-3866.

[109] Cruz, DN; Ronco, C. Acute kidney injury in the intensive care unit: current trends in incidence and outcome. *Crit Care*, 2007, 11, 149.

[110] Chawla, LS; Amdur, RL; Amodeo, S; Kimmel, PL; Palant, CE. The severity of acute kidney injury predicts progression to chronic kidney disease. *Kidney Int.*, 2011 Jun, 79(12), 1361-9.

[111] Parikh, CR; Devarajan, P; Zappitelli, M; Sint, K; Thiessen-Philbrook, H; Li, S; Kim, RW; Koyner, JL; Coca, SG; Edelstein, CL; Shlipak, MG; Garg, AX; Krawczeski, CD. TRIBE-AKI Consortium. Postoperative bio-markers predict acute kidney injury and poor outcomes after pediatric cardiac surgery. *J Am Soc Nephrol*, 2011, 22, 1737-1747.

[112] Bennett, M; Dent, CL; Ma, Q; Dastrala, S; Grenier, F; Workman, R; Syed, H; Ali, S; Barasch, J; Devarajan, P. Urine NGAL predicts severity of acute kidney injury after cardiac surgery: a prospective study. *Clin J Am Soc Nephrol*, 2008, 3, 665-673.

[113] Liangos, O; Tighiouart, H; Perianayagam, MC; Kolyada, A; Han, WK; Wald, R; Bonventre, JV; Jaber, BL. Comparative analysis of urinary bio-markers for early detection of acute kidney injury following cardiopulmonary bypass. *bio-markers*, 2009, 14, 423-431.

[114] Koyner, JL; Vaidya, VS; Bennett, MR; Ma, Q; Worcester, E; Akhter, SA; Raman, J; Jeevanandam, V; O'Connor, MF; Devarajan, P; Bonventre, JV; Murray, PT. Urinary bio-markers in the clinical prognosis and early detection of acute kidney injury. *Clin J Am Soc Nephrol*, 2010, 5, 2154-2165.

[115] Endre, ZH; Pickering, JW; Walker, RJ; Devarajan, P; Edelstein, CL; Bonventre, JV; Frampton, CM; Bennett, MR; Ma, Q; Sabbisetti, VS; Vaidya, VS; Walcher, AM; Shaw, GM; Henderson, SJ; Nejat, M; Schollum, JB; George, PM. Improved performance of urinary bio-markers of acute kidney injury in the critically ill by stratification for injury duration and baseline renal function. *Kidney Int*, 2011, 79, 1119-1130.

[116] Siew, ED; Ikizler, TA; Gebretsadik, T; Shintani, A; Wickersham, N; Bossert, F; Peterson, JF; Parikh, CR; May, AK; Ware, LB. Elevated urinary IL-18 levels at the time of ICU admission predict adverse clinical outcomes. *Clin J Am Soc Nephrol*, 2010, 5, 1497-1505.

[117] Singer, E; Elger, A; Elitok, S; Kettritz, R; Nickolas, TL; Barasch, J; Luft, FC; Schmidt-Ott, KM. Urinary neutrophil gelatinase-associated lipocalin distinguishes pre-renal from intrinsic renal failure and predicts outcomes. *Kidney Int.*, 2011 Aug, 80(4), 405-14.

[118] Perazella MA; Coca, SG; Hall, IE; Iyanam, U; Koraishy, M; Parikh, CR. Urine microscopy is associated with severity and worsening of acute

kidney injury in hospitalized patients. *Clin J Am Soc Nephrol*, 2010, 5, 402-408.

[119] Hall, IE; Coca, SG; Perazella, MA; Eko, UU; Luciano, RL; Peter, PR; Han, WK; Parikh, CR. Risk of poor outcomes with novel and traditional bio-markers at clinical AKI diagnosis. *Clin J Am Soc Nephrol*, 2011, 6, 2740-2749.

[120] Perazella, MA; Coca, SG. Traditional urinary bio-markers in the assessment of hospital-acquired AKI. *Clin J Am Soc Nephrol*, 2012, 7, 167-174.

[121] Macedo, E; Malhotra, R; Bouchard, J; Wynn, SK; Mehta, RL. Oliguria is an early predictor of higher mortality in critically ill patients. *Kidney Int.*, 2011 Oct, 80(7), 760-7.

[122] Cruz, DN; de Cal, M; Garzotto, F; Perazella, MA; Lentini, P; Corradi, V; Piccinni, P; Ronco, C. Plasma neutrophil gelatinase-associated lipocalin is an early biomarker for acute kidney injury in an adult ICU population. *Intensive Care Med*, 2010, 36, 444-451.

[123] de Geus, HR; Bakker, J; Lesaffre, EM; le Noble, JL. Neutrophil gelatinase-associated lipocalin at ICU admission predicts for acute kidney injury in adult patients. *Am J Respir Crit Care Med.*, 2011 Apr 1, 183(7), 907-14.

[124] Kümpers, P; Hafer, C; Lukasz, A; Lichtinghagen, R; Brand, K; Fliser, D; Faulhaber-Walter, R; Kielstein, JT. Serum neutrophil gelatinase-associated lipocalin at inception of renal replacement therapy predicts survival in critically ill patients with acute kidney injury. *Crit Care.*, 2010, 14(1), R9.

[125] Haase, M; Bellomo, R; Devarajan, P; Ma, Q; Bennett, MR; Möckel, M; Matalanis, G; Dragun, D; Haase-Fielitz, A. Novel bio-markers early predict the severity of acute kidney injury after cardiac surgery in adults. *Ann Thorac Surg.*, 2009 Jul, 88(1), 124-30.

[126] Herget-Rosenthal, S; Marggraf, G; Hüsing, J; Göring, F; Pietruck, F; Janssen, O; Philipp, T; Kribben, A. Early detection of acute renal failure by serum cystatin C. *Kidney Int.*, 2004 Sep, 66(3), 1115-22.

[127] Perianayagam, MC; Seabra, VF; Tighiouart, H; Liangos, O; Jaber, BL. Serum cystatin C for prediction of dialysis requirement or death in acute kidney injury: a comparative study. *Am J Kidney Dis*, 2009, 54, 1025-1033.

[128] Nejat, M; Pickering, JW; Walker, RJ; Endre, ZH. Rapid detection of acute kidney injury by plasma cystatin C in the intensive care unit. *Nephrol Dial Transplant*, 2010, 25, 3283-3289.

[129] Seabra, VF; Balk, EM; Liangos, O; Sosa, MA; Cendoroglo, M; Jaber, BL. Timing of renal replacement therapy initiation in acute renal failure: a meta-analysis. *Am J Kidney Dis*, 2008, 52, 272-284.
[130] Cruz, DN; de Geus, HR; Bagshaw, SM. Biomarker strategies to predict need for renal replacement therapy in acute kidney injury. *Semin Dial*, 2011, 24, 124-131.
[131] Srisawat, N; Wen, X; Lee, M; Kong, L; Elder, M; Carter, M; Unruh, M; Finkel, K; Vijayan, A; Ramkumar, M; Paganini, E; Singbartl, K; Palevsky, PM; Kellum, JA. Urinary bio-markers and renal recovery in critically ill patients with renal support. *Clin J Am Soc Nephrol*, 2011, 6, 1815-1823.
[132] Maisel, AS; Mueller, C; Fitzgerald, R; Brikhan, R; Hiestand, BC; Iqbal, N; Clopton, P; van Veldhuisen, DJ. Prognostic utility of plasma neutrophil gelatinase-associated lipocalin in patients with acute heart failure: the NGAL EvaLuation Along with B-type NaTriuretic Peptide in acutely decompensated heart failure (GALLANT) trial. *Eur J Heart Fail*, 2011, 13, 846-851.
[133] Liangos, O; Perianayagam, MC; Vaidya, VS; Han, WK; Wald, R; Tighiouart, H; MacKinnon, RW; Li, L; Balakrishnan, VS; Pereira, BJ; Bonventre, JV; Jaber, BL. Urinary N-acetyl-beta-(D)-glucosaminidase activity and kidney injury molecule-1 level are associated with adverse outcomes in acute renal failure. *J Am Soc Nephrol*, 2007, 18, 904-912.
[134] Siew, ED; Ware, LB; Ikizler, TA. Biological markers of acute kidney injury. *J Am Soc Nephrol*, 2011, 22, 810-820.
[135] McIlroy, DR; Wagener, G; Lee, HT. Neutrophil gelatinase-associated lipocalin and acute kidney injury after cardiac surgery: the effect of baseline renal function on diagnostic performance. *Clin J Am Soc Nephrol*, 2010, 5, 211-219.
[136] Paragas, N; Qiu, A; Zhang, Q; Samstein, B; Deng, SX; Schmidt-Ott, KM; Viltard, M; Yu, W; Forster, CS; Gong, G; Liu, Y; Kulkarni, R; Mori, K; Kalandadze, A; Ratner, AJ; Devarajan, P; Landry, DW; D'Agati, V; Lin, CS; Barasch, J. The Ngal reporter mouse detects the response of the kidney to injury in real time. *Nat Med*, 2011, 17, 216-222.
[137] Eagan, TM; Damås, JK; Ueland, T; Voll-Aanerud, M; Mollnes, TE; Hardie, JA; Bakke, PS; Aukrust, P. Neutrophil gelatinase-associated lipocalin: a biomarker in COPD. *Chest*, 2010, 138, 888-895.
[138] Martí, J; Fuster, J; Hotter, G; Solà, AM; Deulofeu, R; Modolo, MM; Loera, MA; Ferrer, J; Fondevila, C; García-Valdecasas, JC. Serum

neutrophil gelatinase-associated lipocalin in patients with colorectal liver metastases: preliminary results of an exploratory prospective study. *Int J Biol Markers*, 2010, 25, 21-26.

[139] Parikh, CR; Abraham, E; Ancukiewicz, M; Edelstein, CL. Urine IL-18 is an early diagnostic marker for acute kidney injury and predicts mortality in the intensive care unit. *J Am Soc Nephrol*, 2005, 16, 3046-3052.

[140] Lachmann, RA; Werchan, S; Schachtrup, C; Haitsma, JJ; Spener, F; Lachmann, B. Liver-type fatty acid binding protein in serum and broncho-alveolar lavage in a model of acute respiratory failure because of surfactant depletion--a possible marker for lung damage? *Clin Physiol Funct Imaging.*, 2006 Nov, 26(6), 371-5.

[141] Mårtensson, J; Bell, M; Oldner, A; Xu, S; Venge, P; Martling, CR. Neutrophil gelatinase-associated lipocalin in adult septic patients with and without acute kidney injury. *Intensive Care Med*, 2010, 36, 1333-1340.

[142] Washburn, KK; Zappitelli, M; Arikan, AA; Loftis, L; Yalavarthy, R; Parikh, CR; Edelstein, CL; Goldstein, SL. Urinary interleukin-18 is an acute kidney injury biomarker in critically ill children. *Nephrol Dial Transplant*, 2008, 23, 566-572.

[143] Parikh, CR; Coca, SG; Thiessen-Philbrook, H; Shlipak, MG; Koyner, JL; Wang, Z; Edelstein, CL; Devarajan, P; Patel, UD; Zappitelli, M; Krawczeski, CD; Passik, CS; Swaminathan, M; Garg, AX. TRIBE-AKI Consortium. Postoperative bio-markers predict acute kidney injury and poor outcomes after adult cardiac surgery. *J Am Soc Nephrol*, 2011, 22, 1748-1757.

[144] Parikh, CR; Coca, SG; Thiessen-Philbrook, H; Shlipak, MG; Koyner, JL; Wang, Z; Edelstein, CL; Devarajan, P; Patel, UD; Zappitelli, M; Krawczeski, CD; Passik, CS; Swaminathan, M; Garg, AX. TRIBE-AKI Consortium. Postoperative bio-markers predict acute kidney injury and poor outcomes after adult cardiac surgery. *J Am Soc Nephrol*, 2011, 22, 1748-1757.

[145] Han, WK; Waikar, SS; Johnson, A; Betensky, RA; Dent, CL; Devarajan, P; Bonventre, JV. Urinary bio-markers in the early diagnosis of acute kidney injury. *Kidney Int*, 2008, 73, 863-869.

[146] Haase, M; Bellomo, R; Story, D; Davenport, P; Haase-Fielitz, A. Urinary interleukin-18 does not predict acute kidney injury after adult cardiac surgery: a prospective observational cohort study. *Crit Care*, 2008, 12, R96.

[147] Haase-Fielitz, A; Bellomo, R; Devarajan, P; Story, D; Matalanis, G; Dragun, D; Haase, M. Novel and conventional serum bio-markers predicting acute kidney injury in adult cardiac surgery--a prospective cohort study. *Crit Care Med*, 2009, 37, 553-560.
[148] Haase, M; Bellomo, R; Devarajan, P; Ma, Q; Bennett, MR; Möckel, M; Matalanis, G; Dragun, D; Haase-Fielitz, A. Novel bio-markers early predict the severity of acute kidney injury after cardiac surgery in adults. *Ann Thorac Surg*, 2009, 88, 124-130.
[149] Zappitelli, M; Washburn, KK; Arikan, AA; Loftis, L; Ma, Q; Devarajan, P; Parikh, CR; Goldstein, SL. Urine neutrophil gelatinase-associated lipocalin is an early marker of acute kidney injury in critically ill children: a prospective cohort study. *Crit Care.*, 2007, 11(4), R84.
[150] Prowle, JR; Liu, YL; Licari, E; Bagshaw, SM; Egi, M; Haase, M; Haase-Fielitz, A; Kellum, JA; Cruz, D; Ronco, C; Tsutsui, K; Uchino, S; Bellomo, R. Oliguria as predictive biomarker of acute kidney injury in critically ill patients. *Crit Care.*, 2011 Jul 19, 15(4), R172.
[151] Haase, M; Devarajan, P; Haase-Fielitz, A; Bellomo, R; Cruz, DN; Wagener, G; Krawczeski, CD; Koyner, JL; Murray, P; Zappitelli, M; Goldstein, SL; Makris, K; Ronco, C; Martensson, J; Martling, CR; Venge, P; Siew, E; Ware, LB; Ikizler, TA; Mertens, PR. The outcome of neutrophil gelatinase-associated lipocalin-positive subclinical acute kidney injury: a multicenter pooled analysis of prospective studies. *J Am Coll Cardiol*, 2011, 57, 1752-1761.
[152] Morrow, DA; de Lemos, JA. Benchmarks for the assessment of novel cardiovascular bio-markers. *Circulation*, 2007, 115, 949-952.
[153] Maisel, A. Biomonitoring and biomarker-guided therapy: the next step in heart failure and biomarker research. *J Am Coll Cardiol*, 2011, 58, 1890-1892.
[154] Nickolas, TL; O'Rourke, MJ; Yang, J; Sise, ME; Canetta, PA; Barasch, N; Buchen, C; Khan, F; Mori, K; Giglio, J; Devarajan, P; Barasch, J. Sensitivity and specificity of a single emergency department measurement of urinary neutrophil gelatinase-associated lipocalin for diagnosing acute kidney injury. *Ann Intern Med*, 2008, 148, 810-819.
[155] Shapiro, NI; Trzeciak, S; Hollander, JE; Birkhahn, R; Otero, R; Osborn, TM; Moretti, E; Nguyen, HB; Gunnerson, K; Milzman, D; Gaieski, DF; Goyal, M; Cairns, CB; Kupfer, K; Lee, SW; Rivers, EP. The diagnostic accuracy of plasma neutrophil gelatinase-associated lipocalin in the prediction of acute kidney injury in emergency department patients with suspected sepsis. *Ann Emerg Med*, 2010, 56, 52-59. e.l.

[156] Ponce, D; Zorzenon Cde, P; dos Santos, NY; Balbi, AL. Early nephrology consultation can have an impact on outcome of acute kidney injury patients. *Nephrol Dial Transplant*, 2011, 26, 3202-3206.
[157] Mehta, RL; McDonald, B; Gabbai, F; Pahl, M; Farkas, A; Pascual, MT; Zhuang, S; Kaplan, RM; Chertow, GM. Nephrology consultation in acute renal failure: does timing matter? *Am J Med*, 2002, 113, 456-461.
[158] Balasubramanian, G; Al-Aly, Z; Moiz, A; Rauchman, M; Zhang, Z; Gopalakrishnan, R; Balasubramanian, S; El-Achkar, TM. Early nephrologist involvement in hospital-acquired acute kidney injury: a pilot study. *Am J Kidney Dis*, 2011, 57, 228-234.

In: Acute Kidney Injury
Editor: Erika Pearson
ISBN: 978-1-53610-379-3


*Chapter 2*

# REVISITING OLD BIOMARKERS FOR ACUTE KIDNEY INJURY

***Seung Seok Han*[1] *and Sejoong Kim*[1,2]**
[1]Department of Internal Medicine, Seoul National University
College of Medicine, Seoul, Korea
[2]Department of Internal Medicine,
Seoul National University Bundang Hospital, Gyeonggi-do, Korea

## ABSTRACT

New biomarkers for acute kidney injury (AKI) have been proposed; however, they require further validation for use in routine clinical practice. Older biomarkers that are commonly monitored for other purposes have shown potential for predicting the risk of AKI. Complete blood counts (e.g., white blood cells and their subtypes, hemoglobin, red cell distribution width, and platelet volume) are known to be predictors for AKI; however, the natures of the relationships are different for each marker and may be U-shaped, linear, and non-linear with a threshold level. An electrolyte panel (e.g., sodium, potassium, and bicarbonate) is also predictive of AKI, even though the causal relationship is not validated. The baseline liver panel (e.g., liver enzymes, bilirubin, and albumin) strongly predicts subsequent development of AKI, particularly in patients with liver disease or where the liver has been manipulated. Proteinuria and hematuria are easily measured using the dipstick test and are representative markers of chronic kidney injury. They are also predictors for AKI, although the test's low precision and misclassification bias should be acknowledged. Considering these results, this review suggests that old biomarkers can be interpreted for additional clinical usefulness in the prediction of AKI.

## INTRODUCTION

Acute kidney injury (AKI) is a major health concern because it is associated with increased morbidity and mortality [1]. While therapies for AKI have improved in recent years, the prevalence of this condition is still high and continues to increase [2]. Considering these clinical issues, the appropriate detection and management of risk factors related to AKI are important issues for clinicians managing AKI patients.

Current guidelines recommend the use of two parameters, serum creatinine and urine output for diagnosing AKI [3]. However, there are limitations in that serum creatinine has a low sensitivity and specificity of detection in certain states [4], and urine output may confirm only oliguric AKI, and not non-oliguric AKI. Furthermore, hourly measurement of urine output is not feasible in an outpatient environment [5]. Several new biomarkers have been proposed to facilitate earlier and more precise detection of AKI, including neutrophil gelatinase-associated lipocalin and kidney injury molecule-1 [6, 7]. Nevertheless, these biomarkers are not yet fully validated for use in routine clinical practice. The challenge of clinical utilization of new candidates is attributable to the natural characteristics of AKI, which is a complex disease with various causes. Although the use of one biomarker would be ideal in terms of practical availability and lower costs, current knowledge and the evidence available are not sufficient to accommodate this recommendation. Thus, clinicians refer to several laboratory markers and the patient's conditions for predicting AKI. Amongst those laboratory markers routinely checked for purposes other than identifying AKI, some have been known to correlate with the risk and severity of AKI. Herein, we attempt to review the correlation with AKI and predictive value of these factors (i.e., pre-determined laboratory markers are associated with subsequent AKI development). When these factors are considered together with serum creatinine, urine output, and new biomarkers, they may have a potential for precise prediction of AKI.

## COMPLETE BLOOD COUNTS

A routine laboratory examination is the complete blood count, which includes information regarding white blood cells (WBC) and subtypes (e.g., neutrophils, monocytes, lymphocytes, and eosinophils), hemoglobin, and red blood cell count. The scores grading a patient's general illness are rated poor when WBC counts are higher than normal [8, 9]. Likewise, WBC counts can confer the grade for defining the severity of AKI, as the most important mechanism underlying the development of AKI is inflammation [10]. We previously confirmed the relationship between WBC counts and AKI in critically ill patients [11]. Intriguingly, this relationship was U-shaped, wherein both leukopenia and leukocytosis were responsible for a high risk of AKI. These results suggest that current warnings regarding leukocytosis should be expanded to include leukopenia for predicting AKI. When analyses were performed after stratification by WBC subtypes, neutrophilia, but not neutropenia, showed a tendency toward a high risk of AKI; whereas a reverse trend was shown for lymphocytes and monocytes; eosinophils did not correlate with the risk of AKI. Certain studies investigated the ratio between subtypes (e.g., neutrophils and lymphocytes) and found this to be an additional predictor of AKI [12, 13].

In routine blood tests, hemoglobin (or hematocrit) is regarded as a conventional marker of anemia, and low hemoglobin levels are associated with high morbidity and mortality [14, 15]. Additionally, above-normal levels could be related to susceptibility to certain types of diseases and an even higher risk of mortality [16, 17]. Regarding these results, abnormal hemoglobin levels may also correlate with the risk of AKI, and our previous data further supports this issue [18]. The relationship was shown to be non-linear, and high hemoglobin levels above normal range may not provide an advantage in terms of AKI when compared with levels within a normal range (threshold point was calculated as 10.5 g/dL). This parallels the results of previous correlations found between above-normal hemoglobin levels and poorer outcomes [16, 17]. However, this issue should not be confused with the possible adverse effects of blood transfusion. In this review, we restrict our discussion to the predictive value of hemoglobin, although there are many controversial or undetermined issues regarding the use of blood transfusions.

In addition to the above points, other markers such as red cell distribution width [19, 20] and platelet number [21] have been shown to be prognostic factors of AKI. High values of red cell distribution width conferred a high risk of contrast-induced AKI [19, 20], whereas decreased platelet counts was associated with a high risk of AKI in coronary artery bypass grafting [21]. Nevertheless, these data should be interpreted cautiously, because all of these markers are inter-related through both direct and indirect pathways [22, 23].

## ELECTROLYTE PANEL

The electrolyte panel, including sodium, potassium, chloride, and bicarbonate, provides information regarding their levels or the balance of acid-bases. Kidney is the most important organ controlling electrolytes, and conversely, the functioning of kidney can be affected or damaged by abnormal electrolyte levels [24-26]. Based on this knowledge, previous clinical studies have observed electrolyte imbalance and its association with predicting AKI. Hyponatremia has been shown to observed to correlate well with AKI in various clinical settings [27-29]. This relationship is plausible because hyponatremia increases adverse consequences through several effects such as compromised cardiac contractility, increased insulin resistance, and abnormalities in neuromuscular and brain function [30-33]. In addition, hyponatremia can reflect the presence or severity of several comorbidities [34], which is a possible explanation for the relationship. Our previous analyses confirmed that an increase in osmolar gap is associated with a high risk of contrast-induced AKI [35]. Based on the fact that the osmolar gap is primarily altered by sodium levels, our suggested mechanism of action is that hyponatremia induced by the adverse effects of contrast media may increase the osmolar gap, which consequently reflects AKI. In contrast to the current database on hyponatremia, studies investigating the correlation between baseline hypernatremia and subsequent AKI are scarce. However, previous studies have analyzed cross-sectional results at a single time point, where the patients with AKI had a high coincidence of hypernatremia [36, 37], and these suggest that hypernatremia may be also a risk factor of AKI development.

Abnormal potassium levels are frequently observed in both outpatients and inpatients. Based on anecdotal reports, hypokalemia can be a typical marker of AKI, particularly in rhabdomyolysis [38] and diseases resulting in chronic diarrhea [39, 40]. Hyperkalemia is also easily identified in AKI patients when anti-hypertensive drugs (e.g., angiotensin-converting-enzyme inhibitors or angiotensin receptor blockers) or nonsteroidal anti-inflammatory drugs are used [41, 42]. Nevertheless, the predictive value of potassium for AKI remains unresolved due to a lack of cohort studies [43], and further cohort studies are thus needed to elucidate the predictive role of hypokalemia for AKI.

Several experimental models have revealed that metabolic acidosis aggravates the severity of AKI [44, 45]. Additionally, therapies to reverse acidosis have been used in severe cases with metabolic acidosis [46], although this is dependent on the cause of each disease [47]. Nevertheless, the issue as to whether or not metabolic acidosis predicts AKI has not been thoroughly addressed in previous studies. Considering that metabolic acidosis is a frequent feature of AKI [48, 49], we do anticipate that it plays a predictive role \in the risk of developing AKI.

## LIVER PANEL

The liver can be damaged by several toxins or ischemic injury, similar to the kidney, and thus, the processes leading to liver or kidney injury can occur concurrently underwent or be inter-related [50-52]. Liver enzymes (i.e., aspartate transaminase and alanine transaminase) are typical markers of liver damage. Several studies have reported that these enzyme levels can also be increased in patients with kidney injury. Certain studies have concerned the predictive role of baseline liver enzymes for the subsequent development of AKI [53-57]. Cohort data on liver transplant recipients showed that peak levels of aspartate transaminase were higher in cases with AKI development than in counterpart cases [53, 54]. Another study that focused on patients following liver resection further supported the predictive role of liver enzymes (specifically alanine transaminase in this case) [55]. An as yet unexplored relationship is that between liver enzymes and AKI in patients without dominant hepatic injury or any other liver manipulation. Because the liver and kidneys are interrelated and the kidney marker (i.e., serum creatinine) changes slowly, the liver enzymes may in fact have predictive value for the development of AKI in these patient subsets.

The bilirubin level is generally increased in cases of liver injury, and several studies in the clinical setting have previously shown that the increase in bilirubin level correlates with or predicts AKI [56-60]. However, some studies have concerned beneficial effects of bilirubin as an antioxidant and cytoprotective agent [61, 62]. In this regard, certain cross-sectional studies have found a relationship between high bilirubin levels and low risk for various diseases, such as diabetes and cardiovascular disease [63-65].

Nevertheless, no cohort studies have as yet reported an inverse relationship between bilirubin and risk of AKI.

Serum albumin serves as a marker of liver function, nutrition, inflammation, and oncotic pressure. While the underlying mechanisms are not yet fully determined, the relationship between hypoalbuminemia and the risk of AKI has been documented in observational cohort studies. A meta-analysis of 11 studies showed that the risk of AKI significantly increased with a 1.0 g/dL decrease in albumin, with a pooled odds ratio of 2.34 [66]. In addition to this meta-analysis, the results of other subsequent studies support the predictive role of serum albumin for AKI in cardiac surgery and liver transplantation [67-69], although replacement of albumin-containing fluids remains a contradictory issue [70].

## URINALYSIS

Proteinuria and hematuria are criteria for chronic kidney disease [71]; however, these markers are also predictive of AKI in several clinical settings [72-75]. Proteinuria (or albuminuria) can be measured quantitatively using either the total amount or the ratio of concentration to urine creatinine. Most previously acquired data have confirmed the predictive role of proteinuria, based on these methods [72-74]. Herein, we would like to introduce studies that used the dipstick method, a routine examination that has the advantage of easily and inexpensively screening for both proteinuria and hematuria. A large cohort of 920,985 outpatients examined proteinuria using the dipstick method and found that subsequent risk of admission with AKI was well-stratified by proteinuria (rate ratio 4.4 in the heavy proteinuria group vs. the no proteinuria group) [76]. The predictability of proteinuria measured using this test has also been observed in other clinical settings, such as cases of cardiac surgery [77, 78] and burns [79]. In contrast to proteinuria, hematuria is not usually mentioned in large epidemiological studies, and most studies in the field of AKI have not focused on the role it may play. In this regard, our previous work was the first to determine the relationship between hematuria determined by using the dipstick test and the risk of AKI [75], wherein multivariable-adjusted odds ratios for AKI were 1.58 (1+), 2.63 (2+), and 2.52 (3+ by the dipstick test) when compared with non-hematuria in critically ill patients. However, despite the clinical utility and observed results of the dipstick test, its relatively low precision and subsequent misclassification bias should be noted.

Finally, we have summarized all the results listed above in Table 1.

**Table 1. Studies focusing on old biomarkers in predicting acute kidney injury**

| Categories | Items | Risk factors and characteristics | References |
|---|---|---|---|
| Complete blood count | White blood cell | High and low values (U-shaped relationship with AKI); dependence on the subtypes; the ratio between neutrophil and lymphocyte. | 11-13 |
| | Hemoglobin | Low value (non-linear relationship with AKI); threshold value. | 18 |
| | Red cell distribution width | High value. | 19, 20 |
| | Platelet count | Low value. | 21 |
| Electrolyte panel | Sodium | Hyponatremia and hypernatremia. | 27-29, 36, 37 |
| | Osmolar gap | Increased value attributable to hyponatremia. | 35 |
| | Potassium | Hypokalemia and hyperkalemia. | 39-43 |
| | Bicarbonate | Acidosis. | 48, 49 |
| Liver panel | AST and ALT | High value; primarily observed in liver diseases. | 53-57 |
| | Bilirubin | High value; primarily observed in liver diseases. | 56-60 |
| | Albumin | Hypoalbuminemia | 66-69 |
| Urinalysis (dipstick test) | Proteinuria | Positive value; easy and inexpensive screening; low precision. | 75-79 |
| | Hematuria | Positive value; easy and inexpensive screening; low precision. | 75 |

AKI, acute kidney injury; AST, aspartate transaminase; ALT, alanine transaminase.

## ISSUES FOR CONSIDERATION

While the above results are informative, they must be interpreted and applied to clinical practice cautiously. First, the aforementioned studies are observational in nature, and thus could not prove the causality. Second, some markers are known to be predictive only in certain disease states. For example, an association between increased liver enzyme levels and a high risk of AKI has been confirmed solely in patients with liver disease or those who have undergone liver manipulation. Accordingly, the applicability of each study result to other clinical settings should be ruminated. Third, the use of serum creatinine for defining AKI is an imperfect gold standard, although most studies used this marker. Accordingly, the predictability of old biomarkers mentioned above may be less conclusive, especially under conditions where the sensitivity and specificity of creatinine are significantly decreased (e.g., high muscle mass, tubular secretion, and kidney compensation).

## Conclusion

Various new biomarkers have been proposed and validated in an effort to address the early and precise predictability of AKI. However, none of these have yet been fully established in a clinical practice setting. It is fact that some of these new biomarkers are promising, and the old biomarkers presented here are not very sensitive or specific. Nevertheless, these old biomarkers may be helpful for predicting the risk or severity of AKI should be more elaborated, because these are routinely and easily monitored in routine clinical practice and the serum creatinine is not enough to the current need of clinicians.

## References

[1] Chertow GM, Burdick E, Honour M, Bonventre JV, Bates DW. Acute kidney injury, mortality, length of stay, and costs in hospitalized patients. *J. Am. Soc. Nephrol.* 2005;16(11):3365-70.

[2] Lameire N, Van Biesen W, Vanholder R. The changing epidemiology of acute renal failure. *Nat. Clin. Pract. Nephrol.* 2006;2(7):364-77.

[3] Kidney Disease: Improving Global Outcomes (KDIGO) Acute Kidney Injury Work Group. KDIGO Clinical Practice Guideline for Acute Kidney Injury. *Kidney Int. Suppl.* 2012;2:1-138.

[4] Bosch JP, Saccaggi A, Lauer A, Ronco C, Belledonne M, Glabman S. Renal functional reserve in humans. Effect of protein intake on glomerular filtration rate. *Am. J. Med.* 1983;75(6):943-50.

[5] Han SS, Kang KJ, Kwon SJ, Wang SJ, Shin SH, Oh SW, et al. Additional role of urine output criterion in defining acute kidney injury. *Nephrol. Dial. Transplant* .2012;27(1):161-5.

[6] Mishra J, Ma Q, Prada A, Mitsnefes M, Zahedi K, Yang J, et al. Identification of neutrophil gelatinase-associated lipocalin as a novel

early urinary biomarker for ischemic renal injury. *J. Am. Soc. Nephrol.* 2003;14(10):2534-43.

[7] Han WK, Bailly V, Abichandani R, Thadhani R, Bonventre JV. Kidney Injury Molecule-1 (KIM-1): a novel biomarker for human renal proximal tubule injury. *Kidney Int.* 2002;62(1):237-44.

[8] Knaus WA, Draper EA, Wagner DP, Zimmerman JE. APACHE II: a severity of disease classification system. *Crit. Care Med.* 1985;13(10):818-29.

[9] Moreno RP, Metnitz PG, Almeida E, Jordan B, Bauer P, Campos RA, et al. SAPS 3--From evaluation of the patient to evaluation of the intensive care unit. Part 2: Development of a prognostic model for hospital mortality at ICU admission. *Intensive Care Med* 2005;31(10):1345-55.

[10] Bagshaw SM, George C, Bellomo R, Committee ADM. Early acute kidney injury and sepsis: a multicentre evaluation. *Crit. Care* 2008;12(2):R47.

[11] Han SS, Ahn SY, Ryu J, Baek SH, Kim KI, Chin HJ, et al. U-shape relationship of white blood cells with acute kidney injury and mortality in critically ill patients. *Tohoku J. Exp. Med.* 2014;232(3):177-85.

[12] Kim WH, Park JY, Ok SH, Shin IW, Sohn JT. Association Between the Neutrophil/Lymphocyte Ratio and Acute Kidney Injury After Cardiovascular Surgery: A Retrospective Observational Study. *Medicine* 2015;94(43):e1867.

[13] Yilmaz H, Cakmak M, Inan O, Darcin T, Akcay A. Can neutrophil-lymphocyte ratio be independent risk factor for predicting acute kidney injury in patients with severe sepsis? *Ren. Fail.* 2015;37(2):225-9.

[14] Anand I, McMurray JJ, Whitmore J, Warren M, Pham A, McCamish MA, et al. Anemia and its relationship to clinical outcome in heart failure. *Circulation* 2004;110(2):149-54.

[15] Zakai NA, Katz R, Hirsch C, Shlipak MG, Chaves PH, Newman AB, et al. A prospective study of anemia status, hemoglobin concentration, and mortality in an elderly cohort: the Cardiovascular Health Study. *Arch. Intern. Med.* 2005;165(19):2214-20.

[16] John M, Lange A, Hoernig S, Witt C, Anker SD. Prevalence of anemia in chronic obstructive pulmonary disease: comparison to other chronic diseases. *Int. J. Cardiol.* 2006;111(3):365-70.

[17] Regidor DL, Kopple JD, Kovesdy CP, Kilpatrick RD, McAllister CJ, Aronovitz J, et al. Associations between changes in hemoglobin and administered erythropoiesis-stimulating agent and survival in hemodialysis patients. *J. Am. Soc. Nephrol.* 2006;17(4):1181-91.

[18] Han SS, Baek SH, Ahn SY, Chin HJ, Na KY, Chae DW, et al. Anemia Is a Risk Factor for Acute Kidney Injury and Long-Term Mortality in Critically Ill Patients. *Tohoku J. Exp. Med.* 2015;237(4):287-95.

[19] Akin F, Celik O, Altun I, Ayca B, Ozturk D, Satilmis S, et al. Relation of red cell distribution width to contrast-induced acute kidney injury in patients undergoing a primary percutaneous coronary intervention. *Coron. Artery Dis.* 2015;26(4):289-95.

[20] Mizuno A, Ohde S, Nishizaki Y, Komatsu Y, Niwa K. Additional value of the red blood cell distribution width to the Mehran risk score for predicting contrast-induced acute kidney injury in patients with ST-elevation acute myocardial infarction. *J. Cardiol.* 2015;66(1):41-5.

[21] Kertai MD, Zhou S, Karhausen JA, Cooter M, Jooste E, Li YJ, et al. Platelet Counts, Acute Kidney Injury, and Mortality after Coronary Artery Bypass Grafting Surgery. *Anesthesiology* 2016;124(2):339-52.

[22] Roy CN. Anemia of inflammation. *Hematology Am. Soc. Hematol. Educ. Program.* 2010;2010:276-80.

[23] Stokes KY, Granger DN. Platelets: a critical link between inflammation and microvascular dysfunction. *J. Physiol.* 2012;590(5):1023-34.

[24] Kovesdy CP. Significance of hypo- and hypernatremia in chronic kidney disease. *Nephrol. Dial. Transplant.* 2012;27(3):891-8.

[25] Schwartz WB, Relman AS. Effects of electrolyte disorders on renal structure and function. *N. Engl. J. Med.* 1967;276(7):383-9 contd.

[26] Kovesdy CP. Metabolic acidosis and kidney disease: does bicarbonate therapy slow the progression of CKD? *Nephrol. Dial. Transplant.* 2012;27(8):3056-62.

[27] Lameire N, Van Biesen W, Vanholder R. Electrolyte disturbances and acute kidney injury in patients with cancer. *Semin. Nephrol.* 2010;30(6):534-47.

[28] Aronson D, Darawsha W, Promyslovsky M, Kaplan M, Abassi Z, Makhoul BF, et al. Hyponatraemia predicts the acute (type 1) cardio-renal syndrome. *Eur. J. Heart Fail.* 2014;16(1):49-55.

[29] Hackworth WA, Heuman DM, Sanyal AJ, Fisher RA, Sterling RK, Luketic VA, et al. Effect of hyponatraemia on outcomes following orthotopic liver transplantation. *Liver Int.* 2009;29(7):1071-7.

[30] Kozeny GA, Murdock DK, Euler DE, Hano JE, Scanlon PJ, Bansal VK, et al. In vivo effects of acute changes in osmolality and sodium concentration on myocardial contractility. *Am. Heart. J.* 1985;109(2):290-6.

[31] Bratusch-Marrain PR, DeFronzo RA. Impairment of insulin-mediated glucose metabolism by hyperosmolality in man. *Diabetes* 1983;32(11):1028-34.

[32] Knochel JP. Neuromuscular manifestations of electrolyte disorders. *Am. J. Med.* 1982;72(3):521-35.

[33] Aranyi Z, Kovacs T, Szirmai I, Vastagh I. Reversible nerve conduction slowing in hyponatremia. *J. Neurol.* 2004;251(12):1532-3.

[34] Chawla A, Sterns RH, Nigwekar SU, Cappuccio JD. Mortality and serum sodium: do patients die from or with hyponatremia? *Clin. J. Am. Soc. Nephrol.* 2011;6(5):960-5.

[35] Kim S, Sung J, Kang WC, Ahn SY, Kim DK, Chin HJ, et al. Increased plasma osmolar gap is predictive of contrast-induced acute kidney injury. *Tohoku J. Exp. Med.* 2012;228(2):109-17.

[36] Stelfox HT, Ahmed SB, Khandwala F, Zygun D, Shahpori R, Laupland K. The epidemiology of intensive care unit-acquired hyponatraemia and hypernatraemia in medical-surgical intensive care units. *Crit. Care* 2008;12(6):R162.

[37] Kumar AB, Shi Y, Shotwell MS, Richards J, Ehrenfeld JM. Hypernatremia is a significant risk factor for acute kidney injury after subarachnoid hemorrhage: a retrospective analysis. *Neurocrit. Care* 2015;22(2):184-91.

[38] Bosch X, Poch E, Grau JM. Rhabdomyolysis and acute kidney injury. *N Engl. J. Med.* 2009;361(1):62-72.

[39] Menahem SA, Perry GJ, Dowling J, Thomson NM. Hypokalaemia-induced acute renal failure. *Nephrol. Dial. Transplant.* 1999;14(9):2216-8.

[40] Lee EY, Yoon H, Yi JH, Jung WY, Han SW, Kim HJ. Does hypokalemia contribute to acute kidney injury in chronic laxative abuse? *Kidney Res. Clin. Pract.* 2015;34(2):109-12.

[41] Pearce CJ, Gonzalez FM, Wallin JD. Renal failure and hyperkalemia associated with ketorolac tromethamine. *Arch. Intern. Med.* 1993;153(8):1000-2.

[42] Harel Z, Gilbert C, Wald R, Bell C, Perl J, Juurlink D, et al. The effect of combination treatment with aliskiren and blockers of the renin-angiotensin system on hyperkalaemia and acute kidney injury: systematic review and meta-analysis. *BMJ* 2012;344:e42.

[43] Najafi I, Van Biesen W, Sharifi A, Hoseini M, Rashid Farokhi F, Sanadgol H, et al. Early detection of patients at high risk for acute

kidney injury during disasters: development of a scoring system based on the Bam earthquake experience. *J. Nephrol.* 2008;21(5):776-82.

[44] Bank N, Better OS. Acid-base balance and acute renal failure. *Miner. Electrolyte Metab.* 1991;17(2):116-23.

[45] Magalhaes PA, de Brito TS, Freire RS, da Silva MT, Dos Santos AA, Vale ML, et al. Metabolic acidosis aggravates experimental acute kidney injury. *Life Sci.* 2016;146:58-65.

[46] Sabatini S, Kurtzman NA. Bicarbonate therapy in severe metabolic acidosis. *J. Am. Soc. Nephrol.* 2009;20(4):692-5.

[47] Cooper DJ, Worthley LI. Adverse haemodynamic effects of sodium bicarbonate in metabolic acidosis. *Intensive Care Med.* 1987;13(6):425-7.

[48] Rocktaeschel J, Morimatsu H, Uchino S, Goldsmith D, Poustie S, Story D, et al. Acid-base status of critically ill patients with acute renal failure: analysis based on Stewart-Figge methodology. *Crit. Care* 2003;7(4):R60.

[49] de Brito-Ashurst I, Varagunam M, Raftery MJ, Yaqoob MM. Bicarbonate supplementation slows progression of CKD and improves nutritional status. *J. Am. Soc. Nephrol.* 2009;20(9):2075-84.

[50] Epstein M. Hepatorenal syndrome: emerging perspectives of pathophysiology and therapy. *J. Am. Soc. Nephrol.* 1994;4(10):1735-53.

[51] Kelly KJ. Distant effects of experimental renal ischemia/reperfusion injury. *J. Am. Soc. Nephrol.* 2003;14(6):1549-58.

[52] Gardner DS, De Brot S, Dunford LJ, Grau-Roma L, Welham SJ, Fallman R, et al. Remote effects of acute kidney injury in a porcine model. *Am. J. Physiol. Renal Physiol.* 2016;310(4):F259-71.

[53] Leithead JA, Armstrong MJ, Corbett C, Andrew M, Kothari C, Gunson BK, et al. Hepatic ischemia reperfusion injury is associated with acute kidney injury following donation after brain death liver transplantation. *Transpl. Int.* 2013;26(11):1116-25.

[54] Leithead JA, Tariciotti L, Gunson B, Holt A, Isaac J, Mirza DF, et al. Donation after cardiac death liver transplant recipients have an increased frequency of acute kidney injury. *Am. J. Transplant.* 2012;12(4):965-75.

[55] Slankamenac K, Breitenstein S, Held U, Beck-Schimmer B, Puhan MA, Clavien PA. Development and validation of a prediction score for postoperative acute renal failure following liver resection. *Ann. Surg.* 2009;250(5):720-8.

[56] Daher EF, Silva GB, Jr., Karbage NN, Carvalho PC, Jr., Kataoka RS, Silva EC, et al. Predictors of oliguric acute kidney injury in

leptospirosis. A retrospective study on 196 consecutive patients. *Nephron. Clin. Pract* .2009;112(1):c25-30.

[57] Wu CC, Yeung LK, Tsai WS, Tseng CF, Chu P, Huang TY, et al. Incidence and factors predictive of acute renal failure in patients with advanced liver cirrhosis. *Clin. Nephrol.* 2006;65(1):28-33.

[58] Uettwiller-Geiger DL, Vijayendran R, Kellum JA, Fitzgerald RL. Analytical characteristics of a biomarker-based risk assessment test for acute kidney injury (AKI). *Clin. Chim. Acta* 2016;455:93-8.

[59] Uchino S. Outcome prediction for patients with acute kidney injury. *Nephron Clin. Pract.* 2008;109(4):c217-23.

[60] Lima EQ, Zanetta DM, Castro I, Massarollo PC, Mies S, Machado MM, et al. Risk factors for development of acute renal failure after liver transplantation. *Ren. Fail.* 2003;25(4):553-60.

[61] Stocker R, Yamamoto Y, McDonagh AF, Glazer AN, Ames BN. Bilirubin is an antioxidant of possible physiological importance. *Science* 1987;235(4792):1043-6.

[62] Baranano DE, Rao M, Ferris CD, Snyder SH. Biliverdin reductase: a major physiologic cytoprotectant. *Proc. Natl. Acad. Sci. USA* 2002;99(25):16093-8.

[63] Han SS, Na KY, Chae DW, Kim YS, Kim S, Chin HJ. High serum bilirubin is associated with the reduced risk of diabetes mellitus and diabetic nephropathy. *Tohoku J. Exp. Med.* 2010;221(2):133-40.

[64] Kimm H, Yun JE, Jo J, Jee SH. Low serum bilirubin level as an independent predictor of stroke incidence: a prospective study in Korean men and women. *Stroke* 2009;40(11):3422-7.

[65] Perlstein TS, Pande RL, Beckman JA, Creager MA. Serum total bilirubin level and prevalent lower-extremity peripheral arterial disease: National Health and Nutrition Examination Survey (NHANES) 1999 to 2004. *Arterioscler. Thromb. Vasc. Biol.* 2008;28(1):166-72.

[66] Wiedermann CJ, Wiedermann W, Joannidis M. Hypoalbuminemia and acute kidney injury: a meta-analysis of observational clinical studies. *Intensive Care Med.* 2010;36(10):1657-65.

[67] Lee EH, Baek SH, Chin JH, Choi DK, Son HJ, Kim WJ, et al. Preoperative hypoalbuminemia is a major risk factor for acute kidney injury following off-pump coronary artery bypass surgery. *Intensive Care Med* 2012;38(9):1478-86.

[68] Kim WH, Park MH, Kim HJ, Lim HY, Shim HS, Sohn JT, et al. Potentially modifiable risk factors for acute kidney injury after surgery

on the thoracic aorta: a propensity score matched case-control study. *Medicine* 2015;94(2):e273.

[69] Sang BH, Bang JY, Song JG, Hwang GS. Hypoalbuminemia Within Two Postoperative Days Is an Independent Risk Factor for Acute Kidney Injury Following Living Donor Liver Transplantation: A Propensity Score Analysis of 998 Consecutive Patients. *Crit. Care Med.* 2015;43(12):2552-61.

[70] Frenette AJ, Bouchard J, Bernier P, Charbonneau A, Nguyen LT, Rioux JP, et al. Albumin administration is associated with acute kidney injury in cardiac surgery: a propensity score analysis. *Crit. Care* 2014;18(6):602.

[71] Kidney Disease: Improving Global Outcomes (KDIGO) CKD Work Group. KDIGO 2012 Clinical Practice Guideline for the Evaluation and Management of Chronic Kidney Disease. *Kidney Int. Suppl.* 2013;3(1):1-150.

[72] Grams ME, Astor BC, Bash LD, Matsushita K, Wang Y, Coresh J. Albuminuria and estimated glomerular filtration rate independently associate with acute kidney injury. *J. Am. Soc. Nephrol.* 2010;21(10):1757-64.

[73] Koyner JL, Garg AX, Coca SG, Sint K, Thiessen-Philbrook H, Patel UD, et al. Biomarkers predict progression of acute kidney injury after cardiac surgery. *J. Am. Soc. Nephrol.* 2012;23(5):905-14.

[74] Grams ME, Sang Y, Ballew SH, Gansevoort RT, Kimm H, Kovesdy CP, et al. A Meta-analysis of the Association of Estimated GFR, Albuminuria, Age, Race, and Sex With Acute Kidney Injury. *Am. J. Kidney Dis.* 2015;66(4):591-601.

[75] Han SS, Ahn SY, Ryu J, Baek SH, Chin HJ, Na KY, et al. Proteinuria and hematuria are associated with acute kidney injury and mortality in critically ill patients: a retrospective observational study. *BMC Nephrol.* 2014;15:93.

[76] James MT, Hemmelgarn BR, Wiebe N, Pannu N, Manns BJ, Klarenbach SW, et al. Glomerular filtration rate, proteinuria, and the incidence and consequences of acute kidney injury: a cohort study. *Lancet* 2010;376(9758):2096-103.

[77] Huang TM, Wu VC, Young GH, Lin YF, Shiao CC, Wu PC, et al. Preoperative proteinuria predicts adverse renal outcomes after coronary artery bypass grafting. *J. Am. Soc. Nephrol.* 2011;22(1):156-63.

[78] Coca SG, Jammalamadaka D, Sint K, Thiessen Philbrook H, Shlipak MG, Zappitelli M, et al. Preoperative proteinuria predicts acute kidney injury in patients undergoing cardiac surgery. *J. Thorac. Cardiovasc. Surg.* 2012;143(2):495-502.

[79] Hu JY, Meng XC, Han J, Xiang F, Fang YD, Wu J, et al. Relation between proteinuria and acute kidney injury in patients with severe burns. *Crit. Care* 2012;16(5):R172.

In: Acute Kidney Injury
Editor: Erika Pearson

ISBN: 978-1-53610-379-3


*Chapter 3*

# ACUTE KIDNEY INJURY AND NEPHROTOXIC ANTIBIOTIC TREATMENT

***Nadezda Petejova* and Arnost Martinek***

[1]Department of Internal Medicine,
University Hospital Ostrava, Czech Republic
[2]Department of Clinical Studies, Faculty of Medicine,
University of Ostrava, Czech Republic

## ABSTRACT

Acute kidney injury (AKI) is common in clinical settings and an independent predictor of mortality in critically ill patients.

Thus, prevention and early detection of compromised renal function based on serum creatinine levels, urinary output and urinary/serum biomarkers are routinely used in clinical practice. However, appropriate antibiotic treatment is the best lifesaving option in almost all cases of sepsis. Antibiotic treatment is of paramount importance in critically ill septic patients with/without renal damage but a major problem is the necessity for antibiotic drugs with known nephrotoxicity and effects on renal function. In patients with renal replacement and consequently altered antibiotic elimination dynamics, this is of particular relevance. On the other hand, of antibiotic efficacy is reduced if the treatment is not

* Corresponding author: Department of Internal Medicine, University Hospital Ostrava, 17. listopadu, 1790, 708 52 Ostrava, Czech Republic & Department of Clinical Studies, Faculty of Medicine, University of Ostrava, Czech Republic. E-mail: petejova@seznam.cz.

sufficiently controlled. Therapeutic drug monitoring is the most appropriate method for treating septic patients with AKI and for optimising antimicrobial drug serum concentrations without worsening renal function.

**Keywords:** acute kidney injury, antibiotics, nephrotoxic, biomarkers

## Introduction

Acute kidney injury (AKI) is one of the most serious complications in critically ill patients and an independent predictor of mortality. Generally, AKI is presented as a syndrome with rapid decline in kidney function characterized by increase in serum creatinine and/or decrease in urinary output [4]. The incidence of AKI increases with age: in 80 year old critically ill patients, it occurs in 45% [29]. Further, around 6% of all AKI patients require renal replacement therapy with mortality as high as 80% [45]. Patient mortality increases with the severity of AKI disease classified, according to recent KDIGO (Kidney Disease Improving Global Outcome 2012) recommendations into three stages depending on creatinine increase and decrease in diuresis [19]. The general incidence of sepsis induced AKI in hospitalized patients, ranges from 16-25% even in those with milder disease [26]. The results of a multicentre retrospective evaluation of 120,123 patients admitted to general intensive care units (ICU), 33,375 had a sepsis related diagnosis (27.8%). Among septic patients, 14,039 (42.1%) had concomitant AKI (septic AKI) [2]. However, sepsis frequently develops after AKI and portends a poor prognosis, with high mortality rates and relatively long length of hospital stay. Sepsis can be a cause and consequence of AKI depending on oliguria, high fluid accumulation and severity of illness scores, non – surgical procedures after AKI and provision of dialysis [25]. Appropriate antibiotic (ATB) therapy is usually the lifesaving approach in the case of sepsis but with a caveat on serious toxic side effects.

Overall, AKI development in critically ill septic patients has a complex pathophysiology. Further, AKI is not a single disease but rather a syndrome comprising multiple clinical conditions. Outcomes are influenced by the underlying disease causing the condition, as well as by the severity and duration of renal impairment and by the baseline condition of the patient.

## Antibiotic Therapy and the Pathophysiology of Drug-Induced Nephrotoxicity

Drug induced nephrotoxicity is a common complication in hospitalized patients with undesired deterioration in the patient's clinical status and increased economic cost of treating it.

The majority of hospital-acquired AKI cases are due to either prerenal AKI or acute tubular necrosis (ATN); however, unrecognized acute interstitial nephritis (AIN) is likely the third most common cause. In fact, AKI without any obvious cause is found from biopsy-proven AIN to be anywhere from 10 to 27% of patients [35].

Antibiotic or other drug induced nephrotoxicity has become a serious health and economic problem. Antibiotics are one class of antimicrobials drugs. These are divided into two groups depending on their mode of action: 1) bacteriostatic and 2) bactericidal. The differences are based on retarding bacterial growth or killing bacteria. The pharmacokinetic (PK) and pharmacodynamic (PD) profiles of an antimicrobial agent provide key information for helping to establish an efficient dosing regimen. According to PK/PD parameters ATB are divided into three groups [36],[37]:

1. $C_{max}$/MIC dependent ATB – the ratio of the maximum serum concentration of ATB to minimum inhibitory concentration of pathogen; ATB can exhibit a significant post antibiotic effect (e.g., aminoglycosides, fluoroquinolones)
2. T>MIC dependent ATB – the time for which an ATB serum concentration remains above minimum inhibitory concentration of pathogen (e.g.,betalactams, carbapenems)
3. $AUC_{0\text{-}24}$/MIC dependent ATB – the ratio of the area under the serum concentration time curve of ATB during a 24-hour time period to minimum inhibitory concentration of pathogen (vancomycin, tetracyclines, linezolid)

The side effects of an antibiotic can occur under normal dosing regimens and physiological serum concentrations. Typical clinical manifestations of side effects are allergies, dyspepsia, vomiting and indigestion. Acute renal injury mostly associated with antibiotic side effects is acute tubulointerstitial nephritis (AIN). In almost every case, this is a very serious condition characterised by fever, rash, eosinophilia and varying decline of renal function. Urinalysis may reveal microscopic haematuria, proteinuria (often less <1.0g/24 hours) and eosinophils. However, the combination of fever, rash, and eosinophilia for AIN, is a triad only seen in 5 – 10% of patients with AIN [8,35].

Other patterns of tubulointerstitial injury may occur such as Fanconi syndrome, salt-wasting nephropathy, distal renal tubular acidosis and urinary concentrating defects [35].

Antibiotics are also well-established etiology of granulomatous interstitial nephritis (GIN), and the number of implicated agents has grown over time (Table 1). Typically, granulomas exhibit more widespread interstitial infiltration and involve the cortex more than the medulla. Drug-induced AIN is most likely related to an immune reaction as few patients exposed to a particular drug develop AIN. The response is not dose dependent and it can be associated with extrarenal signs of hypersensitivity [39]. However, it is not only drugs that cause GIN. Clinicians must be aware of conditions linked to tuberculosis, sarcoidosis and Wegener's granulomatosis. On renal biopsy, granulomas with non-necrotizing features are associated with drug-induced GIN and sarcoidosis, whereas, necrotizing granulomas are common in patients with granulomatosis with polyangiitis, fungal or tuberculosis-induced GIN [39].

The proximal tubule of the kidney plays a crucial role in renal handling of drugs (e.g., antibiotics, antivirals, diuretics), uremic toxins (e.g., indoxylsulfate), environmental toxins (e.g., mercury, uranium, cadmium, aristolochic acid), metabolites (e.g., uric acid), dietary compounds, and signaling molecules [27]. Organic ion transporters as a consequence, are collectively called multispecific drug transporters. The role of drug transporters in proximal tubule metabolism, raises some interesting questions in the context of renal ischemia and other types of injury (e.g., sepsis). The proximal tubule does require substrates and coupling organic anion transporter (OAT) transport with a-ketoglutarate as the intracellular counter-transporting molecule and plays a role in regulating intracellular levels of citric acid cycle molecules involved in oxidative metabolism. It is not known, at this time whether changes in net proximal tubule OAT activity as a result of altered expression levels or competing anions could affect proximal tubular metabolism and its ability to maintain normal oxidative substrate supply when proximal tubule dynamics are altered due to age, stress, injury or recovery from injury [28].

**Table 1. Type of renal injury due to antibiotic nephrotoxicity [9],[39],[44]**

| Type of acute kidney injury | Antibiotic agent |
|---|---|
| Acute interstitial nephritis | Cephalosporins |
| | Quinolones |
| | Betalactams |
| | Penicillins |
| | Macrolides |
| | Tetracyclines |
| | Lincomycin |
| | Rifampin |
| Granulomatous interstitial nephritis | Vancomycin |
| | Penicillins |
| | Nitrofurantoin |
| | Quinolones |
| | Cephalosporins |
| Acute tubular necrosis | Aminoglycosides |
| | Polymyxins |
| | Vancomycin |
| | Polyene macrolides |
| Crystal nephropathy | Sulfonamides |
| | Quinolones |

The most common nephrotoxic antimicrobials are aminoglycosides, glycopeptides, polymyxins and polyene macrolides. Polypeptide antibiotics such as polymyxins, and aminoglycosides, are essential for treating life-threatening Gram-negative infections. The glycopeptidic antibiotic agent - vancomycin is still used in the treatment of severe Gram-positive infections, especially methicillin - resistant *Staphylococcus aureus.* Polyene macrolides are clinically important antifungal agents often used to treat systemic fungal infections. However, mostly dose-dependent acute kidney injury with acute tubular toxicity attributed to treatment with these agents severely limits their clinical application [9].

In these circumstances, the complexity of the pathophysiology of AKI in septic patients must be emphasised. This progressives with sepsis from systemic inflammatory response syndrome to septic shock. The first problem is the redistribution of corticomedullar renal blood flow following interstitial inflammation, glomerular and tubular injury. The most vulnerable are the proximal tubular cells due to lack of adenosine triphosphate with the development of necrosis [44]. Into this increased pathological process enters the second potential source of kidney injury – nephrotoxic antibiotics. The question is how to treat the severe life-threatening infection obviating secondary renal damage. The issue is confounded due to the combination of sepsis effects on renal parenchyma, the development of septic acute kidney injury and antibiotic nephrotoxicity (Figure 1).

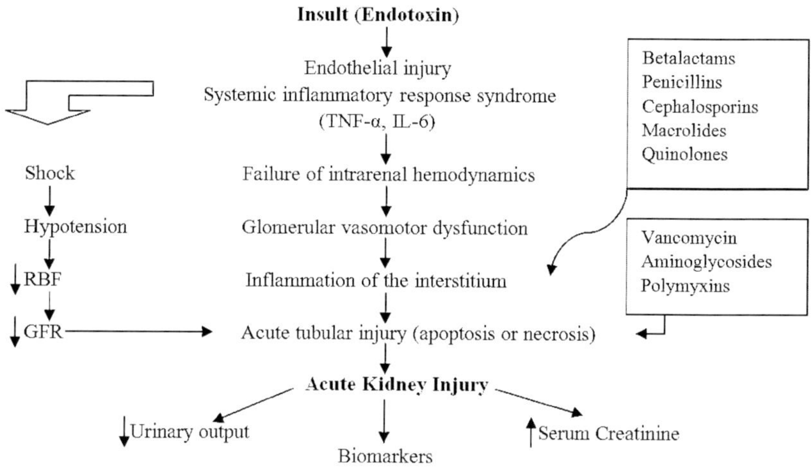


**GFR** – Glomerular Filtration Rate, **IL-6 -** Interleukin - 6, **RBF** – Renal Blood Flow, **TNF-α-** Tumor Necrosis Factor - alpha

Figure. 1. Schematic illustration of AKI development in septic patients and antibiotic nephrotoxicity [9],[13][16],[22],[23],[44].

## Potential Biomarkers of Antibiotic Induced Nephrotoxicity

Given that acute kidney injury is a clinical status with high morbidity and mortality in the setting of both sepsis and nephrotoxicity related to antibacterial treatment, it is of paramount importance to detect an early urinary or serum biomarker of AKI. A number of cytokines, proteins and "omics" have been investigated in this case with varying results and recommendations. The distinction between septic and nephrotoxic AKI in critically ill septic patients, may not be relevant to physicians. However, early recognition of any type of AKI is a key step to the best clinical approach for prevention and protection of the kidney. Serum creatinine is currently used to the greatest extent but this is a poor marker of early renal dysfunction. It is greatly influenced by muscle mass and tubular secretion and can be low in the elderly. Apart from creatinine's adverse effects, comprehensive AKI diagnostics and therapeutic measures according to KDIGO guidelines are based on serum creatinine and urinary output measures [19].

Biomarkers are quantifiable indicators of normal and pathogenic biological processes and pharmacological responses to a therapeutic intervention. They have been introduced in recent years into clinical practise for risk assessment, diagnosis and prognosis of various diseases [5]. One marker of proximal tubular cell injury due to hypoxic conditions causing disruption of megalin dependent endocytosis is Neutrophil Gelatinase-Associated Lipocalin (NGAL). NGAL is a ubiquitous protein comprising 178 amino acids with a molecular mass of around 25 kDa and composed of 8 beta sheets that form a structure [30]. In cases of suspected sepsis, the sensitivity of NGAL has been demonstrated for diagnostic and staging purposes. Plasma NGAL significantly better associates with the renal subscore of the Sequential Organ Failure Assessment in critically ill patients with suspected sepsis than serum creatitine [21],[38]. However, urinary and plasma NGAL is a potential biomarker for many types of AKI without differentiation between nephrotoxic and other types. Another potential biomarker - Kidney Injury Molecule -1 (KIM-1) is a type 1 cell membrane glycoprotein with transmembrane, cytoplasmic and ectodomains. KIM-1 is upregulated in ischemia, nephrotoxic drug injury, chronic kidney disease and decreased kidney transplant function[3]. Vanin-1, an epithelial glycosylphosphatidylinositol-anchored pantetheinase, is invoIed in the response to oxidative stress and has been investigated as a potential biomarker in gentamicin induced nephrotoxicity in animals [14].

Scientific investigation of cell cycle arrest AKI biomarkers, has revealed two possible urine biomarkers for early detection of different types of AKI: 1) TIMP-2 –tissue inhibitor of metalloproteinases-2 and 2) IGFBP7- insulin-like growth factor-binding protein 7. Both markers, TIMP-2 and IGFBP7, are involved in $G_1$ cell cycle arrest in the initial phases of tubular cell injury. TIMP-2 and IGFBP7 are also known to be involved in the response to a wide variety of insults (inflammation, oxidative stress, ultraviolet radiation, drugs and toxins) [15,18].

Biomarkers of acute kidney injury related to treatment with very nephrotoxic antibiotics – aminoglycosides, glycopeptides and polymyxins - have been mostly investigated in animal studies. Little data is available in humans. Potential biomarkers useful in early AKI detection in cases of nephrotoxic antibiotic treatment are summarised in Table 2.

**Table 2. Biomarkers of antibiotic induced nephrotoxicity**

| Antibiotic agent | Urinary biomarkers |
|---|---|
| | (animal studies) |
| Gentamicin | NGAL [17] |
| | Vanin-1 [14] |
| | KIM-1 [46] |
| Vancomycin | KIM-1 [46] |
| Colistin | KIM-1, αGST [20] |

**αGST** – Alpha - Glutathione S-tranferase, **KIM-1** – Kidney Injury Molecule -1, **NGAL** - Neutrophil Gelatinase-Associated Lipocalin

No biomarker is specific to injury caused by any one type of antimicrobial agent and biomarkers can be detected in serum or urine in cases of ischemic/septic injury alone. Hence it is necessary to find more specific "markers" of antibiotic induced AKI. KIM-1 is a notable alternative with high sensitivity and success in predicting drug-induced nephrotoxicity although it is mostly expressed in the proximal tubule, in contrast to the predominant distal convoluted tubule injury found in mice treated with colistin[10].

## Changes in the Pharmacokinetics of Antibiotics in Critically Ill Patients with Acute Kidney Injury

The essential pharmacokinetic parameters of antibiotic agents which can be affected by impaired renal function are: clearance (Cl), volume of distribution (Vd), elimination half-life ($t_{1/2}$), maximum serum concentration ($C_{max}$) and minimum (trough) serum concentration ($C_{min}$)[36]. Clearance is the volume of plasma cleared of the amount of drug excreted per unit of time.With the progressive decline in renal function, there is decreased clearance of hydrophilic, renal eliminated ATB and increase in serum concentration with potentially toxic effects on other organs not only the kidney. Apart from renal elimination of hydrophilic drugs, the liver is the second main elimination route especially in the metabolism of lipophilic drugs [11]. The first step in antimicrobial treatment of patients with AKI is knowledge of type of ATB clearance-via the kidney or the liver. In ATB with predominantly hepatic elimination, no change in dosage regimen is usually required. However in ATB with renal type elimination, it is necessary to change or decrease the dosage. In critically ill septic patients key information is that the loading dose ($D_L$) of antibiotics does not need to be changed and usually can be calculated according to the following equation:

$$D_L = Vd \times C$$ [7], [24]

where C is the targeted ATB serum concentration and Vd is the volume of distribution of ATB. Especially in hydrophilic or renally eliminated drugs, the Vd can be significantly altered and increased due to interstitial capillary leak of fluid or decrease in urinary output in AKI. Further, the elimination half-life can be significantly prolonged with potential development of drug toxicity The maintenance dose depends on ATB clearance and this decreases with elimination organ failure – kidney or liver [11].

The situation is confounded by renal replacement therapy (RRT).

## The Effect of Renal Replacement Therapy on Antibiotic Serum Concentration

Renal replacement therapy is usually used for the treatment of renal failure of either acute or chronic etiology. Intermittent hemodialysis works on the physical principle of the diffusion of solutes through the semipermeable membrane allowing passage mainly of low-molecular weight substances and fluid ultrafiltration. Continuous RRT (CRRT) can operate on other principles outside dialysis. Secondary elimination principles are convection and adsorption at the membrane surface. Many antibiotic agents are small molecular substances with low molecular weight of less than 750 Da, the only exceptions being vancomycin (1,448 Da) and teicoplanin (2,000 Da). These can be removed during dialysis or convection [11,12]. However, eliminate ability is affected by the hydrophilic or lipophilic features of the antimicrobials. Lipophilic antimicrobials usually have high volume of distribution, higher serum protein binding, good intracellular penetration and are metabolised in hepatic elimination. However, hydrophilic agents have a low volume of distribution, lower serum protein binding, poor intracellular penetration and are metabolised by renal elimination [24],[37]]. Based on these facts, it can be assumed that hydrophilic and renally eliminated antimicrobials can be substantially removed by RRT. Further, the extent of drug removal will be determined by other factors: 1) patient clinical status, 2) properties of antimicrobials and 3) characteristics of extracorporeal elimination treatment (Table 3).

**Table 3. The causes of pharmacokinetic changes in antimicrobials during RRT in critically ill septic patients with AKI [7], [33], [36], [40]**

| | |
|---|---|
| Patient's clinical status | Sepsis → severe sepsis → septic shock, Immunological status Age, Body weight, Comorbidity |
| Drug properties | Molecular weight, Lipophility or Hydrophility, Serum Protein Binding, Intracellular penetration, Volume of distribution, Clearance and Metabolism |
| Characteristics of RRT | Type of RRT, Physical principle (diffusion, filtration, adsorption), Type of membrane used and surface area, the pore size of the membrane, Filtration flow rate, Dialysate flow rate, Blood flow rate, Sc and Sd coefficient |

**RRT** – Renal Replacement Therapy, **Sd** – Saturation coefficient, **Sc**- Sieving coefficient

The loading dose of ATB in patients with AKI and RRT does not require changes, while the maintenance dose depends on RRT and non-RRT clearance that can be calculated as:

$$Cl_{ATB}= Cl_{RRT}+ Cl_{non\text{-}RRT} (Cl_{renal} + Cl_{hepatic})$$

In patients with AKI and significant decrease in renal function there can be part hepatic clearance e.g in vancomycin [6]. Clearance of antibiotic agent during intermittent hemodialysis can be calculated according to the following equation:

$$Cl_{ATB}= Cl_{urea} x\ 60/\text{Molecular weight of ATB}$$

where $Cl_{urea}$ is 150 mL/min [41].

Clearance of ATB during continuous renal replacement therapy ($Cl_{CRRT}$) is more complex. The most comprehensive equations for calculating $Cl_{CRRT}$ depending on method, and for calculating a maintenance dose, were established by Choi et al.[7].

In calculating the maintenance dose it is important to know the PK/PD target:

- $C_{max}$/MIC dependent ATB - calculate $t_{1/2} = 0.693xVd/Cl_{tot}$; calculate time to trough ATB concentration and repeat the dose; ($Cl_{tot}$ is a total ATB clearance)
- T>MIC dependent ATB - calculate the maintenance infusion rate from: C x $Cl_{tot}$ (C-is a targeted serum concentration of ATB);
- $AUC_{0-24}$/MIC dependent ATB - calculate target mean serum concentration ($C_p$): target $AUC_{0-24}/24$; and calculate dosing interval: Dose/ ($C_p$ x $Cl_{tot}$); and repeat the loading dose according to calculated dosing interval [7].

However, as mentioned above, patient clinical status can change during over time and typically presents with instability and other coincident parameters then change. The most appropriate way of treating severe infections in septic patients with AKI, necessitating use highly nephrotoxic antibiotics and avoid subtherapeutic serum concentrations - is therapeutic drug monitoring.

## Examples of Therapeutic Drug Monitoring of Dose Dependent Nephrotoxic Antibiotic Treatment in Septic Patients with AKI

***Vancomycin***

Vancomycin is, as mentioned, a glycopeptidic antibiotic agent and is an integral part of empirical treatment in patients with the risk of infection caused by methicilin resistant Ggram-positive groups such as *MRSA*, coagulase-negative S*taphylococci*, *Enterococcus faecium*, or therapy targeted at these pathogens [43].

## Pharmacokinetics/Pharmacodynamics Parameters

Vancomycin is administered intravenously for the treatment of systemic infections but is poorly absorbed after oral administration. The apparent Vd in steady state is reported to be 0.39 (up to 0.9) L/kg. Vancomycin is bound to plasma proteins by 30 to 55% and even higher and in the human organism it is poorly metabolized. Following parenteral administration, it is excreted almost completely as a microbiologically active substance (approx. 70-80% within 24 hours) through glomerular filtration via the kidneys. Biliary excretion is insignificant (less than 5% of a dose) [43]. Hepatic clearance around 16 mL/min (range 3.8-23.3 mL/min) contributes significantly to Vancomycin elimination in patients with AKI [6].

In patients with normal renal function the serum half-life is about 4-6 (5-11) hours, in children 2.2-3.0 hours. In cases of impaired renal function, the half-life of vancomycin may be considerably prolonged (up to 7.5 days) [43]. Vancomycin is a time – and $AUC_{0\text{-}24}$/MIC dependent antibiotic. Critically ill patients with impaired renal function and treated by any form of renal replacement therapy are at high risk of treatment failure due to subtherapeutic serum concentration or at risk of developing acute tubular necrosis. The loading dose in critically ill septic patients is not reduced irrespective of renal function the same as for patients without AKI, or calculated from desire serum concentration multiplied by volume of distribution. The recommended daily intravenous dose is 2,000 mg (2g), divided into 500 mg doses administered every 6 hours or (1g) 1,000 mg every 12 hours in adults patients. Each dose should be administered at no more than 10 mg/min or over a period of at least 60 minutes. In patients with impaired renal function, the maintenance dose should be adjusted according to renal function. Troughs should be obtained just prior to the next dose under vancomycin steady-state conditions (just before the fourth dose) [1].

## Assay and Dose Adjustement Regimens

Serum and ultrafiltrate vancomycin concentrations are determined using fluorescence polarisation immunoassay as the most appropriate for clinical TDM. Vancomycin maintenance dose adjustment can be made via simulation using an appropriate pharmacokinetics programme. Dose adjustment can be made by proportionally increasing or decreasing the dose relative to the target concentration and AUC/MIC ratio. The targeted vancomycin trough serum concentration is 10-20 mg/L and for severe infections or continuous administration of 20-25 mg/L [47]. An AUC/MIC ratio of ≥400, has been advocated as a target to achieve clinical efficacy. However, as it can be difficult in the clinical setting to obtain multiple serum vancomycin concentrations to determine AUC and then calculate AUC/MIC, trough serum concentration monitoring, which can be used as a surrogate marker for AUC, is recommended as the most accurate and most practical method for vancomycin monitoring [1].

## Sampling Time in Critically Ill Patients with AKI and Treated by Daily Intermittent Hemodialysis

Vancomycin can be significantly removed during hemodialysis and better is application after the procedure or in the last hour of dialysis. Due to high pharmacokinetic variability in acute septic patients with AKI, daily monitoring of vancomycin serum concentrations before the next dialysis is optimal. During the 3-6 h following dialysis, blood concentrations of vancomycin can signifficantly rebound, reflecting a vancomycin redistribution phase [6]. Following cessation of dialysis, blood levels rise as vancomycin equilibrates from tissue to blood. Consequently, estimates of vancomycin removal based on immediate post-dialysis serum levels will overestimate its dialytic clearance.Thus, it might also be appropriate to monitor vancomycin serum concentration 6-12 hours after dialysis and before the next dialysis [32].

## Sampling Time in Critically Ill Patients with AKI and Treated by CRRT

Due to the unstable patient clinical status and possible fluctuations in RRT, daily monitoring of vancomycin serum levels is necessary, at least for the first few days after antibiotic introduction. Achievement of adequate vancomycin concentration on the first day of treatment in septic patients is of the utmost clinical importance. Recommended is blood sampling as early as 6 hour after first vancomycin dose in case of the need for early dose adjustment or in the interval 6-12 hours after the first dose [31].

### *Gentamicin*

Gentamicin is an aminoglycoside antibiotic agent effective in the treatment of Gram-negative infections. Gentamicin is bactericidal in action, concentration dependent with substantial postantibiotic effect. This can prevent bacterial regrowth for prolonged periods should drug concentrations fall below the minimum inhibitory concentration [36]. Although the exact mechanism of action has not been fully elucidated, the drug appears to inhibit protein synthesis in susceptible bacteria by irreversibly binding to 30S ribosomal subunits. In general, gentamicin is active against many aerobic Gram-negative bacteria and some aerobic Gram-positive bacteria [42].

## Pharmacokinetics/Pharmacodynamics Parameters

Binding of aminoglycoside antibiotics to blood plasma proteins is low, less than 10%. For this reason, elimination of gentamicin using appropriate methods can be significant and lead to decreased gentamicin blood levels. The Vd of gentamicin is about equivalent to the volume of extracellular water. In the newborn, water comprises 70 to 75% of bodyweight, compared with 50 to 55% in adults. The extracellular water compartment is larger- 40% of body weight compared with 25% of body weight in adults [42]. Gentamicin is not metabolised in the human body and is eliminated via glomerular filtration. The daily dose recommended in children, adolescents and adults with normal renal function, is 3-6 mg/kg body weight per day as 1 (preferred) up to 2 single doses. Dosage is adjusted for patients with renal impairment to minimise the risk of toxicity and the dosing interval according to KDIGO recommendation for AKI patients is every 24 hours. The most important nephrotoxicity and ototoxicity are related to the total dose [19].

## Assay and Dose Adjustment Regimens

Serum and ultrafiltrate gentamicin concentrations are best determined using fluorescence polarisation immunoassay and analysed using a pharmacokinetic programme. To optimise gentamicin treatment efficacy in critically ill patients, extended – interval dosing with $C_{max}$ monitoring and MIC determination of the pathogen is the most appropriate practice [36]. The optimal peak concentration is $C_{max}$/MIC ratio 8–10, but not greater than 14 mg/L and trough concentration less than 2 mg/L (the potential toxicity thresholds)[6],[37].

## Sampling Time in Patients with AKI and Treated by Intermittent Daily Hemodialysis

Gentamicin can be removed during hemodialysis and most appropriate is application before the procedure to imitate its physiological pharmacokinetics and to avoid the development of nephrotoxicity.

To achieve a steady state concentration of antibiotic, it is necessary to maintain the drug elimination. Due to high pharmacokinetic variability, in acute septic patients with AKI daily monitoring of gentamicin serum concentrations, 30-60 min after application and after 24 hours (before the next dose) is optimal. However, the daily dialysis regimen may not lead to decrease of $C_{min}$ below the targeted concentration of 2 mg/L with potential risk of nephrotoxicity. One possible option in this situation is to prolong the dosing interval beyond 24 hours or time of dialysis procedure [33]

## Sampling Time in Patients with AKI and Treated by CRRT

Due to unstable clinical status and possible fluctuations in RRT, daily monitoring of gentamicin serum levels is necessary at least for the first few days after antibiotic introduction. CRRT in critically ill patients can lead to rapid high and consistent extracorporeal removal of gentamicin and total clearence can approach normal renal function. However, we should bear in mind that CRRT cessation would lead to a decrease in total clearance with the possibility of drug accumulation. The dose of gentamicin and/or dosage interval should be adequately adjusted to minimize the risk of toxicity. Recommended is blood sampling 30-60 min after application and after 24 hours or before the next dose [34].

# Conclusion

Knowledge of the contribution of renal replacement therapy to antibiotic clearance could facilitate achieving the right antibiotic dose for optimal antibiotic activity and minimising potential toxicity. The exact differentiation between septic and nephrotoxic AKI in critically ill septic patients has less clinical importance. However both pathophysiological processes substantially contribute to patient outcome and can increase mortality. On the other hand, subtherapeutic serum antibiotic concentrations are unacceptable especially in severe sepsis. For this reason, therapeutic monitoring of antibiotic serum concentrations, if available, is a valuable tool in drug dosage adjustment.

The project was supported by grant of Ministry of Health Czech Republic IGA MZCR NS 10309–3/2009.

# References

[1] American Society of Health-System Pharmacists. Therapeutic monitoring of vancomycin in adult patients: A consensus review of the American Society of Health-System Pharmacists, the Infectious Diseases Society of America, and the Society of Infectious Diseases Pharmacists. (2009). *Am. J. Health-Syst. Pharm.*, *66*, 82–98.

[2] Bagshaw, S.M., George, C. and Bellomo, R. (2008). ANZICS Database Management Committee. Early acute kidney injury and sepsis: a multicentre evaluation. Crit. Care[On-line serial]12. http://ccforum. com/ content/ 12/2/R47.

[3] Belcher, J.M.,Edelstein, C.L. and Parikh, C.R. (2011). Clinical applications of biomarkers for acute kidney injury. *Am. J. Kidney. Dis.*, *57*, 930-940.

[4] Bellomo, R., Kellum, J.A. &Ronco, C. (2012). Acute kidney injury. *Lancet.*, *380*, 756-766.

[5] Bonicolini, E., Romagnoli, S., De Gaudio, A.F. &Petrin, F. (2013). Biomarkers in organ failure. *Trends in Anaesthesia and Critical Care*, *3*, 97-104.

[6] Burton, M. E., Shaw, L. M.,Scheritag, J. J., Evans, V.E. (2006). *Applied Pharmacokinetics and Pharmacodynamics Principles of Therapeutic Drug Monitoring*; 4th Edition. Philadelphia, PA: Lippincote Williams and Wilkins.

[7] Choi, G., Gomersall, C.D., Tian, Q., Joynt, G.M., Freebairn, R. &Lipman, J. (2009). Principles of antibacterial dosing in continuous renal replacement therapy.*Crit. Care. Med.*,*37*, 2268-2282.

[8] Clarkson, M.R., Giblin, L., O'Connell, F.P., O'Kelly, P., Walshe, J.J., Conlon, P., O'Meara, Y., Dormon, A., Campbell, E. &Donohoe, J. (2004). Acute interstitial nephritis: clinical features and response to corticosteroid therapy. *Nephrol. Dial. Transplant.*, *19*, 2778-2783.

[9] De Pont, A.-C. J. M., Prowle, J. R., Legrand, M.Groeneveld, A. B. J. (2015). Etiology and Pathophysiology of Acute Kidney Injury. In: Oudemans-van Straaten HM, Forni LG, Groeneveld, ABJ, Bagshaw SM, Joannidis M editors. *Acute Nephrology for the Critical Care Physician*. Springer Cham Heidelberg New York Dordrecht London:Springer International Publishing, pp. 39-56.

[10] Eadon, M.T., Hack, B.K., Alexander, J.J., Xu, C., Dolan, M.E. and Cunningham, P.N. (2013). Cell cycle arrest in a model of colistin nephrotoxicity. *Physiol. Genomics*, *45*, 877-888.

[11] Eyler, R.F. and Mueller, B.A. (2011). Antibiotic dosing in critically ill patients with acute kidney injury. *Nat. Rev. Nephrol.*, *7*, 226-235.

[12] Glossop, A.& Seidel, J. (2008). Dosing regimes for antimicrobials during continuous veno-venous haemofiltration (CVVH). *Journal of the Intensive Care Society* [On-line serial], 9 (2). http:// inc.sagepub. com/ content /9 /2/ 160. full.pdf+html.

[13] Honore, P.M., Jacobs, R., Hendrickx, I., Bagshaw, S.M., Joannes - Boyau, O., Boer, W., De Waele, E., Van Gorp,V. and Spapen, H.D. (2015). Prevention and treatment of sepsis-induced acute kidney injury: an update. *Ann. Intensive. Care*, *5*, 51.

[14] Hosohata, K., Ando, H. and Fujimura, A. (2012). Urinary vanin-1 as a novel biomarker for early detection of drug-induced acute kidney injury. *J. Pharmacol. Exp. Ther.*, *341*, 656-662.

[15] Hoste, E.A., McCullough, P.A., Kashani, K., Chawla, L.S., Joannidis, M., Shaw, A.D., Feldkamp, T., Uettwiller-Geiger, D.L., McCarthy, P.,Shi, J., Walker, M.G. and Kellum, J.A., Sapphire Investigators. (2014). Derivation and validation of cutoffs for clinical use of cell cycle arrest biomarkers. *Nephrol. Dial. Transplant*, *29*, 2054-2061.

[16] Jacobs, R., Honore, P.M., Joannes-Boyau, O., Boer. W., De Regt, J., De Waele, E., Collin, V. &Spapen, H. D. (2011). Septic acute kidney injury: the culprit is inflammatory apoptosis rather than ischemic necrosis. *Blood. Purif.*, *32*, 262-265.

[17] Kai, K., Yamaguchi, T.,Yoshimatsu, Y., Kinoshita, J., Teranishi, M. and Takasaki, W. (2013). Neutrophil gelatinase-associated lipocalin, a sensitive urinary biomarker of acute kidney injury in dogs receiving gentamicin. *J. Toxicol. Sci.*, *38*, 269-277.

[18] Kashani, K., Al-Khafaji, A., Ardiles, T., Artigas, A., Bagshaw, S.M., Bell, M., Bihorac, A., Birkhahn, R., Cely, C.M., Chawla, L.S., Davison, D.L., Feldkamp, T., Forni, L.G., Gong, M.N.,Gunnerson, K.J., Haase, M., Hackett, J., Honore, P.M., Hoste, E.A., Joannes-Boyau, O., Joannidis, M., Kim, P., Koyner, J.L., Laskowitz, D.T., Lissauer, M.E., Marx, G.,McCullough, P.A., Mullaney, S., Ostermann, M., Rimmelé, T., Shapiro, N.I., Shaw, A.D., Shi, J., Sprague, A.M., Vincent, J.L., Vinsonneau, C., Wagner, L., Walker, M.G., Wilkerson, R.G.,Zacharowski, K. and Kellum, J.A.(2013). Discovery and validation of cell cycle arrest biomarkers in human acute kidney injury. *Crit. Care* [On-line serial], 17.http:// ccforum. com/content/17/1/R25.

[19] Kidney Disease: Improving Global Outcomes (KDIGO) Acute Kidney Injury Work Group. KDIGO Clinical Practice Guideline for Acute Kidney Injury. (2012). *Kidney Inter. Suppl.*, *2*, 1–138.

[20] Keirstead, N.D., Wagoner, M.P., Bentley, P., Blais, M., Brown, C., Cheatham, L., Ciaccio, P., Dragan, Y., Ferguson, D., Fikes, J., Galvin, M., Gupta, A., Hale, M., Johnson, N., Luo, W., McGrath, F., Pietras, M., Price, S., Sathe, A.G., Sasaki, J.C., Snow, D., Walsky, R.L. and Kern, G. (2014). Early prediction of polymyxin-induced nephrotoxicity with next-generation urinary kidney injury biomarkers. *Toxicol. Sci.*, *137*, 278-291.

[21] Kim, H., Hur, M., Cruz, D.N., Moon, H.W. and Yun, Y.M. (2013). Plasma neutrophil gelatinase-associated lipocalin as a biomarker for acute kidney injury in critically ill patients with suspected sepsis. *Clin. Biochem.*, *46*, 1414-1418.

[22] Lee, D.W., Faubel, S. and Edelstein, C.L. (2011). Cytokines in acute kidney injury (AKI).*Clin. Nephrol.*, *76*, 165-173.

[23] Matejovic, M. (2010). The Kidney in Sepsis. [Ledviny v sepsi]. *Postgradualni medicina.*, *9*, 1042-1047.

[24] McKenzie, C. (2011). Antibiotic dosing in critical illness. *J. Antimicrob. Chemother.*, 66, (suppl 2), 25-31.

[25] Mehta, R.L, Bouchard, J., Soroko, S.B., Ikizler, T.A., Paganini, E.P., Chertow, G.M. &Himmelfarb, J. Program to Improve Care in Acute Renal Disease (PICARD) Study Group. (2011). Sepsis as a cause and consequence of acute kidney injury: Program to Improve Care in Acute Renal Disease. *Intensiv. Care. Med.*, *37*, 241-248.

[26] Mårtensson, J. &Bellomo, R. (2015). Sepsis-Induced Acute Kidney Injury. *Crit. Care. Clin.*, *31*, 649-660.

[27] Nigam, S.K. (2015). What do drug transporters really do? *Nat. Rev. Drug. Discov.*, *14*, 29-44.

[28] Nigam, S.K., Wu, W., Bush, K.T., Hoenig, M.P., Blantz, R.C. &Bhatnagar, V. (2015). Handling of Drugs, Metabolites, and Uremic Toxins by Kidney Proximal Tubule Drug Transporters. *Clin. J. Am. Soc. Nephrol.*, *10*, 2039-2049.

[29] Nisula, S., Kaukonen, K.M., Vaara, S.T., Korhonen, A.M., Poukkanen, M., Karlsson, S., Haapio, M., Inkinen, O., Parviainen, I., Suojaranta-Ylinen, R., Laurila, J.J., Tenhunen, J., Reinikainen, M., Ala-Kokko, T., Ruokonen, E., Kuitunen, A. &Pettilä, V. FINNAKI Study Group. (2013). Incidence, risk factors and 90-day mortality of patients with acute kidney injury in Finnish intensive care units: the FINNAKI study.

*Intensive. Care. Med., 39,* 420-428. Erratum in: *Intensive. Care. Med., 39,* 798.

[30] Noto, A., Cibecchini, F., Fanos, V. &Mussap, M. (2013). NGAL and metabolomics: the single biomarker to reveal the metabolome alterations in kidney injury. Biomed. Res. Int [On-line serial], 2013.http:// dx.doi. org/ 10. 1155/2013/612032.

[31] Petejova, N., Martinek, A., Zahalkova, J., Duricova, J., Brozmannova, H., Urbanek, K., Grundmann, M., Plasek, J. &Kacirova, I. (2014). Vancomycin pharmacokinetics during high-volume continuous venovenous hemofiltration in critically ill septic patients. *Biomed. Pap., 158,*65-72.

[32] Petejova, N., Martinek, A., Zahalkova, J., Duricova, J., Brozmanova, H., Urbanek, K., Grundmann, M.&Kacirova, I. (2012). Vancomycin removal during low-flux and high-flux extended daily hemodialysis in critically ill septic patients. *Biomed. Pap., 56,*342-347.

[33] Petejova, N. (2015). [The Antibiotic Treatment in Septic Patients with Acute Kidney Injury treated by Renal Replacement Therapy]. In: Rychlík I, Editor. [*The Future Pharmacotherapy in Nephrology*].Prague: Mladá fronta, 2015, pp. 40-54.

[34] Petejova, N., Zahalkova, J., Duricova, J., Kacirova, I., Brozmanova, H., Urbanek, K., Grundmann, M. &Martinek, A. (2012). Gentamicin pharmacokinetics during continuous venovenous hemofiltration in critically ill septic patients. *J. Chemother., 24,* 107-112.

[35] Perazella, M.A. (2014). Diagnosing drug-induced AIN in the hospitalized patient: a challenge for the clinician. *Clin. Nephrol., 81,* 381-388.

[36] Roberts, J.A.& Lipman, J. (2009).Pharmacokinetic issues for antibiotics in the critically ill patient. *Crit. Care. Med., 37,* 840-851.

[37] Roberts, J.A., Norris, R., Paterson, D.L.& Martin, J.H. (2012). Therapeutic drug monitoring of antimicrobials. *Br. J. Clin. Pharmacol, 73,* 27-36.

[38] Ronco, C. (2014). Biomarkers for acute kidney injury: is NGAL ready for clinical use? *Crit. Care* [On-line serial], 18. http:// ccforum. com/ content/ 18/6/680.

[39] Shah, S., Carter-Monroe, N. and Atta, M.G. (2015). Granulomatous interstitial nephritis. *Clin. Kidney. J., 8,* 516-523.

[40] Schetz, M. (2007). Drug dosing in continuous renal replacement therapy: general rules. *Curr. Opin. Crit. Care, 13,* 645-651.

[41] Sulkova, S., et al., [Hemodialysis]. 1st Edition.Prague, Czech republic: Maxdorf; 2000.
[42] Summary of product characteristics (gentamicin). [online]. 2015 [cited 2016 04 03]. Available from: URL: https:// www. medicines. org.uk/ emc/medicine/21665 - Gentamicin 40 mg/ml Injection - Summary of Product Characteristics (SPC) – (eMC).
[43] Summary of product characteristics (vancomycin). [online]. 2014 [cited 2016 04 03]. Available from: URL: https://www.medicines. org.uk/ emc/ medicine/ 21291 – Vancocin Powder for Solution – Summary of Product Characteristics (SPC) – (eMC).
[44] Teplan, V. [Acute Kidney Injury and Failure in Clinical Medicine]. 1st Edition. Prague, Czech Republic: Grada Publishing a.s; 2010.
[45] Tolwani, A. (2012). Continuous renal-replacement therapy for acute kidney injury. *N. Engl. J. Med.*, *367*, 2505-2514.
[46] Vaidya,V.S., Ozer, J.S., Dieterle, F., Collings, F.B., Ramirez, V., Troth, S., Muniappa, N., Thudium, D., Gerhold, D., Holder, D.J., Bobadilla, N.A., Marrer, E., Perentes, E., Cordier, A., Vonderscher, J., Maurer, G., Goering, P.L., Sistare, F.D. and Bonventre, J.V. (2010). Kidney injury molecule-1 outperforms traditional biomarkers of kidney injury in preclinical biomarker qualification studies. *Nat. Biotechnol.*, *28*, 478-485.
[47] Wong, G., Sime, F.B., Lipman, J.& Roberts, J.A. (2014). How do we use therapeutic drug monitoring to improve outcomes from severe infections in critically ill patients? BMC. Infect. Dis [On-line serial], 14, http:// www. biomedcentral.com/1471-2334/14/288.

## *BIOGRAPHICAL SKETCH*

### *Nadezda Petejova, MD, PhD*

**Affiliation:** Department of Internal Medicine, University Hospital, Ostrava, Czech Republic Department of Clinical Studies, University of Ostrava, Czech Republic

**Education:** 1992 -1998 Faculty of Medicine, Safarik University Kosice, Slovak Republic - M.D.

2001 Study Certificate Grade I in Internal Medicine, Institute for Postgraduate Medical Education, Bratislava, Slovak Republic

2005 Study Certificate Grade II in Internal Medicine, Institute for PostgraduateMedical Education, Prague, Czech Republic

2009 Study Certificate in Nephrology, Institute for Postgraduate Medical Education Prague, Czech Republic

Since 2007 – to 2012 Postgraduate doctoral study Ph.D - Faculty of Medicine Palacky UniversityOlomouc, Czech Republic
*Theme of Doctoral Thesis:*Therapeutic monitoring and changes of pharmacokinetics ofselected antibiotics during continuous and intermittent renal replacement therapy incritically ill septic patients with acute kidney injury

Since 2014 - to present – Postgraduate study: Master of Health Administration (MHA) at St. ElizabethUniversity of Health and Social Sciences in Bratislava, Slovak Republic.
*Theme of diploma thesis:* The management of prevention and treatment of acute kidney injury.

10- 15th March 2014 – Postgraduate Course Attendance: The Update in Medicine–Harvard Medical School, Boston, Massachusetts, USA
13- 20th July 2014 – Postgraduate Course Attendance: The 37th Annual Intensive Review of Internal Medicine (IRIM) Course –Harvard Medical School, Boston, Massachusetts, USA

**Membership in Scientific Societies**

Czech Nephrology Society
Czech Transplant Society
Czech Society of Internal Medicine
European Society of Organ Transplantation

**Research and Professional Experience**

**Grants: as partner**

Since 03/2009 - to 2012 Grant: IGA NS 103 09 - 3/2009 (Ministry of Health Czech Republic):
Changes of pharmacokinetics of vancomycin and gentamicin during continuous and intermitent renal replacement therapy in sepsis and acute kidney injury, the use of predictive pharmacokinetic modeling at dosage of selected antibiotics

Since 2013 – at present Grant: The Institutional support of University Hospital Ostrava n.2 RVO-FNOs/ 2013:
The identification of factors in development acute renal failure in patients with polytrauma
Since 2006 – at present - part-time lecturer at the Medical Faculty of the University of Ostrava
Since 2011 – at present - member of attestation commission of nursing care in anesthesia, resuscitation and intensive care
Since 2012 – at present – part-time lecturer on Crtitical Care Nephrology Courses at the Institute of postgraduate medical education in Prague, Czech Republic

**Professional Appointments:**
**Current position:**
Since 1.5.2003 at present - Senior House Officer, Department of Internal Medicine, University Hospital Ostrava
**Past Positions:**
1998-1999 House Officer, Department of Internal Medicine, Hospital Svidník, Slovak Republic
1999-2003 House Officer, Department of Internal Medicine, Hospital Rimavská Sobota, Slovak Republic

**Honors:**Award of the Czech Nephrology Society for the best publication in 2014.

**Publications Last 3 Years:**

Petejova, N., Martinek, A. (2014) Acute kidney injury due to rhabdomyolysis and renal replacement therapy: a critical review CRITICAL CARE Volume: 18 Issue: 3 Article Number: 224 Published:2014 Times cited: 5 (Scopus), Times cited: 5, IF 4,476 (Web of Science)
Petejova, N., Martinek, A. (2015). Renal cell carcinoma: review of etiology, pathophysiology and risk factors. Biomed.Pap. Med. Fac.Univ.Palacky. Olomouc Czech Repub. 2015; 159: Online 3 nov 2015 (ahead of print): doi.org/10.5507/bp.2015.050. IF 1,200/2015 (review)
Petejova, N., Martinek, A., Zahalkova, J. et al.: Vancomycin pharmacokinetics during high-volume continuous venovenous hemofiltration in critically ill septic patientsBIOMEDICAL PAPERS-OLOMOUC Volume: 158 Issue: 1 Pages: 65-72 Published: 2014 Times Cited: 5, IF – 1,2 (Scopus, Web of Science)

Plasek, J., Doupal, V., Furstova, J. et al.: The role of adrenomedullin and galanin in recurrent vasovagal syncope: a case control studyBIOMEDICAL PAPERS-OLOMOUC Volume: 157 Issue: 2 Pages: 162-167 Published: 2013 Times Cited: 1, IF – 1,2 (Scopus, Web of Science)

Kacirova, I., Petejova, N., Duricova, J.; et al.: Vancomycin Removal During Low-Flux and High-Flux Extended Daily Hemodialysis in Critically Ill Septic Patients. Conference: 13th International Congress of Therapeutic Drug Monitoring and Clinical Toxicology Location: Salt Lake City, UTDate: SEP 22-26, 2013. THERAPEUTIC DRUG MONITORING. Volume: 35.Issue: 5.Pages: 693-694.Published: OCT 2013, IF – 2,234, (Web of Science)

Petejova, N., Martinek, A.: Acute kidney injury following acute pancreatitis: A review. BIOMEDICAL PAPERS-OLOMOUC. Volume: 157.Issue: 2.Pages: 105-113.Published: 2013, IF – 0,990, Times cited: 7 (Scopus), Times cited: 6 (Web of Science)

Petejova, N., Martinek, A., Zahalkova, J., et al. Vancomycin removal during low-flux and high-flux extended daily hemodialysis in critically ill septic patients BIOMEDICAL PAPERS-OLOMOUC Volume: 156 Issue: 4 Pages: 342-347 Published: 2012., IF-0,990, Times cited: 7, (Scopus), Times cited: 5(Web of Science)

Vrkocova, K., Rudolecka, J., Petejova, N., Plevova, P.: [Noncompation cardiomyopathy – a rare cause of heart failure] (2015). Interni Medicina pro Praxi, 17 (1), pp. 31-34. Times cited: 0 (Scopus)

Petejova, N., Martinek, A. [Rhabdomyolysis and acute kidney injury - editorial] – (2014). Vnitr. Lek, 60(3):pp.189-191. Times cited: 0 (PubMed)

Sagan, J., Roznovsky, L., Petejova, N., Mrazek, J., Dankova, D. [Unusual cause of severe Leptospirosis] (2014). Klin. Mikrobiol. Inf. Lék. 20(3): pp. 102-104.

Valkovsky, I., Tvrdik, J., Martinek, A., Olsanska, R., Dedochova, J., Petejova, N., Svagera, Z., Pernicova, M., Cermakova, Z.: [Bone mineral density in patients with chronic renal failure at the start of haemodialysis therapy (2012). Vnitr. Lek., 58 (11), pp. 817-824. Times cited: 1, (Scopus)

Petejova, N., Martinek, A., Zahalkova, J., Duricova, J., Plasek, J., Valkovsky, I., Grundmann, M., Kacirova, I. [An effect of continuous and intermittent renal replacement therapy on antibiotic treatment in critically ill patients with sepsis – A practice-based perspective of vancomycin and gentamicin therapies] (2012). Vnit. Lek, 58 (6), pp. 448-454. Times cited 5. (Scopus)

**Chapters in medical book:**

Petejova, N. (2015) [Acute Kidney Injury in the Elderly]. In: Teplan V editor: [*Nephrology in the Elderly*] Prague: Mladá fronta, pp. 297-314. ISBN 978-80-204-3521-7.

Petejova, N. (2015). [The Antibiotic Treatment in Septic Patients with Acute Kidney Injury treated by Renal Replacement Therapy]. In: Rychlík, I, Editor: [*The Future Pharmacotherapy in Nephrology*]. Prague: Mladá fronta, 2015, pp. 40-54. ISBN 978-80-204-3865-2.

# BIBLIOGRAPHY


**Acute kidney injury: causes, diagnosis, and treatments**

| | |
|---|---|
| *LCCN* | 2011002412 |
| *Type of material* | Book |
| *Main title* | Acute kidney injury: causes, diagnosis, and treatments / Jonathan D. Mendoza, editor. |
| *Published/Created* | New York: Nova Biomedical/Nova Science Publishers, c2011. |
| *Description* | x, 188 p.: ill.; 27 cm. |
| *ISBN* | 9781612097909 (hardcover: alk. paper)<br>1612097901 (hardcover: alk. paper) |
| *LC classification* | RC918.R4 A328 2011 |
| *Related names* | Mendoza, Jonathan D. |
| *Contents* | How to define and classify acute kidney injury (AKI): the risk injury failure loss of kidney function end-stage kidney disease (RIFLE) and acute kidney injury network (AKIN) classifications / José António Lopes, Sofia Jorge -- Acute renal failure in the newborn (NB) / Nilzete Liberato Bresolin -- Kidney ischemia and reperfusion injury / Valquiria Bueno -- Long-term prognostic implication of post-angiographic acute kidney injury and hemodynamic instability / Tomonori Kimura, Yoshitaka Isaka, Terumasa Hayashi -- Cardiac surgery-associated acute diney injury / Vijaykumar Lingegowda, Mourad Alsabbagh and A. Ahsan Ejaz -- Innate and adaptive immune response in |

| | |
|---|---|
| | acute kidney injury: new plays in the play offs! / Mariane Tami Amano ... [et al.] -- Pandemic H1N1 influenza A infection and acute kidney injury / David Collister ... [et al.] -- Biomarkers in acute kidney injury / Michael A. Ferguson, Vishal S. Vaidya, Joseph V. Bonventre -- Sepsis: acute kidney injury and B2 adrenoceptor therapy / Ako Nakamura -- Role of oxidative stress in renal ischemia/reperfusion injury / Satoshi Hagiwara, Hironori Koga and Takayuki Noguchi. |
| *Subjects* | Acute renal failure.<br>Acute Kidney Injury. |
| *Notes* | Includes bibliographical references and index. |
| *Series* | Nephrology research and clinical developments |

**ADQI consensus on AKI biomarkers and cardiorenal syndromes**

| | |
|---|---|
| *LCCN* | 2013010987 |
| *Type of material* | Book |
| *Main title* | ADQI consensus on AKI biomarkers and cardiorenal syndromes / volume editors, Peter A. McCullough, Novi, Mich., John A. Kellum, Pittsburgh, Pa., Ravindra L. Mehta, San Diego, Calif., Patrick T. Murray, Dublin, Claudio Ronco, Vicenza. |
| *Published/Produced* | Basel: Karger, 2013. |
| *Description* | xi, 203 pages: illustratons; 25 cm. |
| *ISBN* | 9783318024067 (hard cover: alk. paper) |
| *LC classification* | RD575 .A29 2013 |
| *Variant title* | Acute Dialysis Quality Initiative consensus on acute kidney injury biomarkers and cardiorenal syndromes |
| *Related names* | McCullough, Peter A., editor of compilation.<br>Kellum, John A., editor of compilation.<br>Mehta, Ravindra L., editor of compilation.<br>Murray, Patrick T., editor of compilation.<br>Ronco, C. (Claudio), 1951- editor of compilation.<br>Acute Dialysis Quality Initiative.<br>Conference on Biomarkers in AKI (10th: 2011: Dublin, Ireland)<br>Conference on CRS (11th: 2012: Venice, Italy) |

*Contents* Acute Dialysis Quality Initiative (ADQI) / Ronco, C., Kellum, J., Bellomo, R., Mehta, R. -- Implementation of novel biomarkers in the diagnosis, prognosis, and management of acute kidney injury: executive summary from the tenth consensus conference of the Acute Dialysis Quality Initiative (ADQI) / McCullough, P.A., for the Acute Dialysis Quality Initiative (ADQI) Consensus Group -- Diagnosis of acute kidney injury using functional and injury biomarkers: workgroup statements from the tenth Acute Dialysis Quality Initiative Consensus Conference / McCullough, P.A., for the ADQI 10 Workgroup -- Differential diagnosis of AKI in clinical practice by functional and damage biomarkers: workgroup statements from the tenth Acute Dialysis Quality Initiative Consensus Conference / Endre, Z.H., for the ADQI 10 Workgroup -- Use of biomarkers to assess prognosis and guide management of patients with acute kidney injury / Cruz, D.N., for the ADQI 10 Workgroup -- Physiological biomarkers of acute kidney injury: a conceptual approach to improving outcomes / Okusa, M.D., for the ADQI 10 Workgroup -- Pathophysiology of the cardiorenal syndromes: executive summary from the eleventh onsensus conference of the Acute Dialysis Quality Initiative (ADQI) / McCullough, P.A., for the Acute Dialysis Quality Initiative (ADQI) Consensus Group -- Pathogenesis of cardiorenal syndrome type 1 in acute decompensated heart failure: workgroup statements from the eleventh consensus conference of the Acute Dialysis Quality Initiative (ADQI) / Haase, M., for the Acute Dialysis Quality Initiative (ADQI) Consensus Group -- Pathophysiology of cardiorenal syndrome type 2 in stable chronic heart failure: workgroup statements from the eleventh consensus conference of the Acute Dialysis Quality Initiative (ADQI) / Cruz, D.N.,; for the Acute Dialysis Quality Initiative (ADQI) Consensus Group -- Cardiorenal syndrome type 3: pathophysiologic and epidemiologic considerations /

| | |
|---|---|
| | Bagshaw, S.M., for the Acute Dialysis Quality Initiative 11 Working Group -- Cardiorenal syndrome type 4: insights on clinical presentation and pathophysiology from the eleventh consensus conference of the Acute Dialysis Quality Initiative (ADQI) / Tumlin, J.A., for the Acute Dialysis Quality Initiative (ADQI) 11 Consensus Group -- Cardiorenal syndrome type 5: clinical presentation, pathophysiology, and management strategies from the eleventh consensus conference of the Acute Dialysis Quality Initiative (ADQI) / Mehta, R.L., for the Acute Dialysis Quality Initiative (ADQI) 11 Working Group. |
| *Subjects* | Acute Kidney Injury--Congresses.<br>Biological Markers--Congresses.<br>Cardio-Renal Syndrome--Congresses. |
| *Notes* | Includes bibliographical references and indexes. |
| *Series* | Contributions to nephrology, 0302-5144; vol. 182<br>Contributions to nephrology; v. 182. 0302-5144 |

**Andreoli and Carpenter's Cecil essentials of medicine**

| | |
|---|---|
| *LCCN* | 2009027158 |
| *Type of material* | Book |
| *Main title* | Andreoli and Carpenter's Cecil essentials of medicine / editor-in-chief, Thomas E. Andreoli; editors, Ivor J. Benjamin, Robert C. Griggs, Edward J. Wing. |
| *Edition* | 8th ed. |
| *Published/Created* | Philadelphia, PA: Saunders/Elsevier, c2010. |
| *Description* | xxvii, 1282 p.: ill. (some col.); 28 cm. |
| *ISBN* | 9781416061090<br>1416061096 |
| *LC classification* | RC46 .C42 2010 |
| *Portion of title* | Cecil essentials of medicine<br>Essentials of medicine |
| *Related names* | Andreoli, Thomas E., 1935-<br>Cecil, Russell L. (Russell La Fayette), 1881-1965. |
| *Contents* | Molecular basis of human disease -- Evidence-based medicine, quality of life, and the cost of medicine -- Structure and function of the normal heart and blood vessels -- Evaluation of the patient with cardiovascular |

disease -- Diagnostic tests and procedures in the patient with cardiovascular disease -- Heart failure and cardiomyopathy -- Congenital heart disease -- Acquired valvular heart disease -- Coronary heart disease -- Cardiac arrhythmias -- Pericardial and myocardial disease -- Other cardiac topics -- Vascular diseases and hypertension -- The lung in health and disease -- General approach to patients with respiratory disorders -- Evaluating lung structure and function -- Obstructive lung diseases -- Interstitial lung diseases -- Pulmonary vascular disease -- Disorders of respiratory control -- Disorders of the pleura, mediastinum, and chest wall -- Infectious diseases of the lung -- Essentials in critical care medicine -- Neoplastic disorders of the lung -- Preoperative and postoperative care -- Elements of renal structure and function -- Approach to the patient with renal disease -- Fluid and electrolyte disorders -- Glomerular diseases -- Major nonglomerular disorders -- Vascular disorders of the kidney -- Acute kidney injury -- Chronic renal failure -- Common clinical manifestations of gastrointestinal disease -- A: Abdominal pain -- B: Gastrointestinal hemorrhage -- C: Malabsorption -- D: Diarrha -- Endoscopic and imaging procedures -- Esophageal disorders -- Diseases of the stomach and duodenum -- Inflammatory bowel disease -- Neoplasms of the gastrointestinal tract -- Diseases of the pancreas -- Laboratory tests in liver disease -- Jaundice -- Acute and chronic hepatitis -- Fulminant hepatic failure -- Cirrhosis of the liver and its complications -- Disorders of the gallbladder and biliary tract -- Hematopoiesis and hematopoietic failure -- Clonal disorders of the hematopoietic stem cell -- Disorders of red blood cells -- Clinical disorders of neutrophils -- Disorders of lymphocytes -- Normal hemostasis -- Disorders of hemostasis: bleeding -- Disorders of hemostasis: thrombosis -- Cancer biology and etiologic factors -- Cancer epidemiology and cancer prevention -- Solid tumors -- Complications of cancer and cancer treatment -- Principles of cancer therapy -- Obesity -- Anorexia nervosa and bulimia nervosa -- Malnutrition, nutritional assessment, and nutritional support in adult patients -- Disorders of lipid metabolism -- Disorders of metals and metalloproteins -- Hypothalamic-pituitary axis -- Thyroid gland -- Adrenal gland -- Male reproductive endocrinology -- Diabetes mellitus -- Hypoglycemia -- Women's health topics -- A: Introduction -- B: Preventive health recommendations for women -- C: Health issues across the life course -- D: Special topics -- Men's health topics -- A: Benign prostatic hyperplasia -- B: Prostatitis -- C: Erectile dysfunction -- D: Carcinomas of men -- E: Benign scrotal diseases -- Normal physiology of bone and mineral homeostasis -- Disorders of serum minerals -- Metabolic bone diseases -- Osteoporosis -- Paget disease of bone -- Approach to the patient with rheumatic disease -- Rheumatoid arthritis -- Spondyloarthropathies -- Systemic lupus erythematosus -- Antiphospholipid antibody syndrome -- Systemic sclerosis (scleroderma) -- Idiopathic inflammatory myopathies -- Sjögrén syndrome -- Systemic vasculitis -- Crystal arthropathies -- Osteoarthritis -- Nonarticular soft tissue disorders -- Rheumatic manifestations of systemic disorders -- Organisms that infect humans -- Host defenses against infection -- Laboratory diagnosis of infectious diseases -- Antimicrobial therapy -- Fever and febrile syndromes -- Bacteremia and sepsis syndrome -- Infections of the nervous system -- Infections of the head and neck -- Infections of the lower respiratory tract -- Infections of the heart and blood vessels -- Skin and soft tissue infections -- Intra-abdominal abscess and peritonitis -- Infectious diarrhea -- Infections involving bones and joints -- Infections of the urinary tract -- Health care-associated infections -- Sexually transmitted infections -- Human immunodeficiency virus infection and acquired immunodeficiency syndrome -- Infections in the immunocompromised

| | |
|---|---|
| | host -- Infectious diseases of travelers: protozoal and helminthic infections -- Bioterrorism -- Neurologic evaluation of the patient -- Disorders of consciousness -- Disorders of sleep -- Cortical syndromes -- Dementia and memory disturbances -- Major disorders of mood, thoughts, and behavior -- Disorders of thermal regulation -- Headache, neck pain, and other painful disorders -- Disorders of vision and hearing -- Dizziness and vertigo -- Disorders of the motor system -- Developmental and neurocutaneous disorders -- Cerebrovascular disease -- Traumatic brain injury and spinal cord injury -- Epilepsy -- Central nervous system tumors -- Infectious diseases of the nervous system -- Demyelinating and inflammatory disorders -- Neuromuscular diseases: disorders of the motor neuron and plexus and peripheral nerve disease -- Muscle diseases -- Neuromuscular junction disease -- The aging patient -- Palliative care -- Alcohol and substance abuse. |
| *Subjects* | Internal medicine--Textbooks.<br>Internal Medicine. |
| *Notes* | Includes bibliographical references and index. |

**Applied therapeutics: the clinical use of drugs.**

| | |
|---|---|
| *LCCN* | 2011047631 |
| *Type of material* | Book |
| *Main title* | Applied therapeutics: the clinical use of drugs. |
| *Edition* | 10th ed. / edited by Brian K. Alldredge ... [et al.]. |
| *Published/Created* | Philadelphia: Wolters Kluwer/Lippincott Williams and Wilkins, c2013. |
| *Description* | xxxix, 2519 p.: ill.; 29 cm. |
| *ISBN* | 9781609137137 (hbk.)<br>1451175760 (hbk.) |
| *LC classification* | RM262 .A65 2013 |
| *Variant title* | Applied therapeutics |
| *Cover title* | Koda-Kimble and Young's applied therapeutics: the clinical use of drugs |
| *Other title* | Koda-Kimble and Young's applied therapeutics: the clinical use of drugs |

| | |
|---|---|
| *Related titles* | Applied therapeutics. |
| *Related names* | Koda-Kimble, Mary Anne.<br>Alldredge, Brian K. |
| *Contents* | Sect. 1: General care -- Assessment of therapy and medication therapy management -- Interpretation of clinical laboratory tests -- Anaphylaxis and drug allergies -- Managing drug overdoses and poisonings -- End-of-life care -- Nausea and vomiting -- Pain and its management -- Perioperative care -- Acid-base disorders -- Fluid and electrolyte disorders -- Vaccinations -- Anemias -- Sect. 2: Cardiac and vascular disorders -- Dyslipidemias, atherosclerosis, and coronary heart disease -- Essential hypertension -- Peripheral vascular disorders -- Thrombosis -- Chronic stable angina -- Acute coronary syndrome -- Heart failure -- Cardiac arrhythmias -- Hypertensive crises -- Shock -- Sect. 3: Pulmonary disorders -- Asthma -- Chronic obstructive pulmonary disease -- Acute and chronic rhinitis -- Cystic fibrosis -- Sect. 4: Gastrointestinal disorders -- Upper gastrointestinal disorders -- Lower gastrointestinal disorders -- Complications of end-stage liver disease -- 505 0 $a Sect. 5: Renal disorders -- Acute kidney injury -- Chronic kidney disease -- Renal dialysis -- Dosing of drugs in renal failure -- Sect. 6: Solid organ transplantation -- Kidney and liver transplantation -- Sect. 7: Nutrition issues -- Basics of nutrition and patient assessment -- Obesity -- Adult enteral nutrition -- Adult parenteral nutrition -- Sect. 8: Dermatologic disorders -- Dermatotherapy and drug induced skin disorders -- Acne -- Psoriasis -- Photosensitivity, photoaging, and burn injuries -- Sect. 9: Arthritic disorders -- Osteoarthritis -- Rheumatoid arthritis -- Gout and hyperuricemia -- Connective tissue disorders -- Sect. 10: Women's health -- Contraception -- Infertility -- Obstetric drug therapy -- Disorders related to the menstrual cycle -- The transition through menopause -- Sect. 11: Endocrine disorders -- Thyroid disorders -- Diabetes mellitus -- Sect. 12: Eye |

disorders -- Eye disorders -- Sect. 13: Neurologic disorders -- Multiple sclerosis -- Headache -- Parkinson disease and other movement disorders -- Seizure disorders -- Cerebrovascular disorders -- Sect. 14: Infectious disorders -- Principles of infectious diseases -- Antimicrobial prophylaxis for surgical procedures -- Central nervous system infections -- Endocarditis -- Respiratory tract infections -- Tuberculosis -- Infectious diarrhea -- Intra-abdominal infections -- Urinary tract infections -- Sexually transmitted diseases -- Osteomyelitis and septic arthritis -- Traumatic skin and soft tissue infections -- Prevention and treatment of infections in neutropenic cancer patients -- Pharmacotherapy of human immunodeficiency virus infection -- Opportunistic infections in HIV-infected patients -- Fungal infections -- Viral infections -- Viral hepatitis -- Parasitic infections -- Tick-borne diseases -- Sect. 15: Psychiatric disorders -- Anxiety disorders -- Sleep disorders -- Schizophrenia -- Mood disorders I: major depressive disorders -- Mood disorders II: bipolar disorder -- Attention deficit hyperactivity disorder in children, adolescents, and adults -- Sect. 16: Substance abuse -- Drug abuse -- Alcohol use disorders -- Tobacco use and dependence -- Sect. 17: Neoplastic disorders -- Neoplastic disorders and their treatment: general principles -- Adverse effects of chemotherapy and targeted agents -- Pediatric malignancies -- Adult hematologic malignancies -- Breast cancer -- Lung cancer -- Colorectal cancer -- Hematopoietic cell transplantation -- Sect. 18: Pediatrics -- Pediatric pharmacotherapy -- Pediatric fluid, electrolytes, and nutrition -- Common pediatric illnesses -- Neonatal therapy -- Care of the critically ill child -- Sect. 19: Geriatric therapy -- Geriatric drug use -- Geriatric dementias -- Geriatric urologic disorders -- Osteoporosis.

*Subjects* Chemotherapy.
Pharmacology.

| | |
|---|---|
| | Chemotherapy--Handbooks, manuals, etc. |
| | Drug Therapy--methods. |
| *Notes* | Rev. ed. of: Applied therapeutics: the clinical use of drugs / edited by Mary Anne Koda-Kimble ... [et al.]. 9th ed. c2009. |
| | Includes bibliographical references and index. |

**Biomarkers: in medicine, drug discovery, and environmental health**

| | |
|---|---|
| *LCCN* | 2010013135 |
| *Type of material* | Book |
| *Main title* | Biomarkers: in medicine, drug discovery, and environmental health / edited by Vishal S. Vaidya, Joseph V. Bonventre. |
| *Published/Created* | Hoboken, N.J.: Wiley, c2010. |
| *Description* | xxviii, 602 p., [16] p. of plates: ill. (some col.); 25 cm. |
| *ISBN* | 9780470452240 (hardback) |
| | 0470452242 (hardback) |
| *LC classification* | QH438.4.B55 B555 2010 |
| *Related names* | Vaidya, Vishal S. |
| | Bonventre, Joseph V. |
| *Summary* | "This book provides an introduction to the field of biomarkers, how they have been and can be used, and how different approaches can be used to identify, characterize, and monitor biomarkers. The book has chapters on topics including HIV, Cancer, Parkinson's, vascular injury, environmental exposure. A following section discusses the technologies (diagnostics and assays) to detect biomarkers and authors have emphasized the preclinical and clinical manifestation of the injury/disease process"--Provided by publisher. |
| *Contents* | Biomarkers: an evolutionary perspective / Michael A. Ferguson and Vishal S. Vaidya -- Genomics / Weida Tong and Donna L. Mendrick -- Proteomics for biomarker discovery / Timothy D. Veenstra -- Metabolic profiling for biomarker discovery / Hector C. Keun -- The bittersweet promise of glycobiology / Padmaparna Chaudhuri, Rania Harfouche, and Shiladitya Sengupta -- Biomarkers of Alzheimer's and Parkinson's disease / Walter Maetzler and Daniela |

Berg -- Biomarkers of cardiac injury / Anthony S. McLean and Stephen J. Huang -- Lung injury biomarkers / Urmila P. Kodavanti -- Translational biomarkers of acute drug-induced liver injury: the current state, gaps, and future opportunities / Josef S. Ozer ... [et al.] -- Biomarkers of acute kidney injury / Frank Dieterle and Frank D. Sistare -- In search of biomarkers for drug-induced vascular injury / James R. Turk -- Biomarkers of immunotoxicity / Rodney R. Dietert -- Biomarkers in obstetric medicine / Manish Maski, Sarosh Rana, and S. Ananth Karumanchi -- Biomarkers in cancer / Roopali Roy ... [et al.] -- Biomarkers of HIV / Lewis Kaufman and Michael J. Ross -- Biomarkers of in vitro drug-induced mitochondrial dysfunction / James A. Dykens and Yvonne Will -- Immunoassay-based technologies for the measurement of biological materials used for biomarkers discovery and translational research / Vincent Ricchiuti -- Nanoscale techniques for biomarker quantification / Madhukar Varshney and Harold G. Craighead -- Immunodiagnostics with a focus on lateral flow point-of-care devices / Roy R. Mondesire ... [et al.] -- Biomarkers for environmental exposure / Jane E. Gallagher, Elaine A. Cohen Hubal, and Stephen W. Edwards -- Clinical study design in biomarker research / Orfeas Liangos and Bertrand L. Jaber -- Statistical issues in biomarker research / Daniel Holder and Matthew Schipper -- Regulatory perspective for biomarker qualification from the U.S. FDA / Federico Goodsaid -- The European Medicines Agency approach / Marisa Papaluca Amati and Spiros Vamvakas.

*Subjects* Biochemical markers.
Biological Markers.
Diagnostic Techniques and Procedures.
Drug Discovery.
Environmental Monitoring--methods.

*Notes* Includes bibliographical references and index.

**Cardiopulmonary bypass**

| | |
|---|---|
| *LCCN* | 2015016868 |
| *Type of material* | Book |
| *Uniform title* | Cardiopulmonary bypass (Ghosh) |
| *Main title* | Cardiopulmonary bypass / edited by Sunit Ghosh, Florian Falter, Albert C. Perrino, Jr. |
| *Edition* | Second edition. |
| *Published/Produced* | Cambridge; New York: Cambridge University Press, 2015. |
| *ISBN* | 9781107428256 (paperback) |
| *LC classification* | RD598 |
| *Related names* | Ghosh, S. (Sunit), editor.<br>Falter, Florian, editor.<br>Perrino, Albert C., Jr., editor. |
| *Contents* | Equipment and monitoring for cardiopulmonary bypass / Victoria Molyneux and Andrew A. Klein -- Cardiopulmonary bypass circuit setup and safety checks / Hannah Kiziltug and Simon Colah -- Priming solutions for cardiopulmonary bypass circuits / Christiana Georgiou and Joanne Irons -- Anticoagulation, coagulopathies, blood transfusion and conservation in cardiac surgery / Liza Enriquez and Linda Shore-Lesserson -- Conduct of cardiopulmonary bypass / Christiana Burt, Saran Hutton and Betsy Evans -- Metabolic management during cardiopulmonary bypass / Kevin Collins and G. Burkhard Mackensen -- Myocardial protection and cardioplegia / Maurice Hogan and David Jenkins -- Weaning from cardiopulmonary bypass / Amy Needham and Christopher P.R. Walker -- Mechanical circulatory support / Kirsty Dempster and Steven Tsui -- Deep hypothermic circulatory arrest / Joseph E. Arrowsmith and Charles W. Hogue -- Organ damage during cardiopulmonary bypass / Christopher C. C. Hudson and Sherif Assaad -- Cerebral morbidity in adult cardiac surgery / David J. Cook and Sean M. Bruggink -- Acute kidney injury (AKI) in cardiac surgery / Robert C. Albright -- Extracorporeal membrane oxygenation / Loreta Grecu -- Paediatric |

| | |
|---|---|
| | aspects of cardiopulmonary bypass / D.D.L. Wong and Craig R. Bailey -- Non-cardiac surgery functions of cardiopulmonary bypass / Lay Ping Ong and Sukumaran K. Nair. |
| *Subjects* | Cardiopulmonary Bypass--methods.<br>Cardiac Surgical Procedures--methods. |
| *Notes* | Includes bibliographical references and index. |

**Critical care medicine: the essentials**

| | |
|---|---|
| *LCCN* | 2009030607 |
| *Type of material* | Book |
| *Personal name* | Marini, John J. |
| *Main title* | Critical care medicine: the essentials / John J. Marini, Arthur P. Wheeler. |
| *Edition* | 4th ed. |
| *Published/Created* | Philadelphia: Wollters Kluwer/Lippincott Williams and Wilkins, c2010. |
| *Description* | xii, 708 p.: ill.; 26 cm. |
| *Links* | Publisher description http://www.loc.gov/catdir/enhancements/fy1010/2009030607-d.html<br>Table of contents only http://www.loc.gov/catdir/enhancements/fy1012/2009030607-t.html |
| *ISBN* | 9780781798396<br>0781798396 |
| *LC classification* | RC86.8 .M386 2010 |
| *Related names* | Wheeler, Arthur P. |
| *Contents* | Hemodynamics -- Hemodynamic monitoring -- Support of the failing circulation -- Arrhythmias, pacing, and cardioversion -- Respiratory monitoring -- Airway intubation -- Indications and options for mechanical ventilation -- Practical problems and complications of mechanical ventilation -- Positive end-expiratory and continuous positive airway pressure -- Weaning and discontinuation of mechanical ventilation -- Intensive care unit imaging -- Acid-base disorders -- Fluid and electrolyte disorders -- Blood conservation and transfusion -- Pharmacotherapy -- Nutritional assessment and support -- Analgesia, sedation, and therapeutic paralysis -- General |

| | |
|---|---|
| | supportive care -- Quality improvement and cost control -- Cardiopulmonary arrest -- Acute coronary syndromes -- Hypertensive emergencies -- Venous thromboembolism -- Oxygenation failure, ARDS, and acute lung injury -- Ventilatory failure -- ICU infections -- Severe sepsis -- Thermal disorders -- Acute kidney injury and renal replacement therapy -- Clotting and bleeding disorders and anticoagulation therapy -- Hepatic failure -- Endocrine emergencies -- Drug overdose and poisoning -- Neurological emergencies -- Chest trauma -- Acute abdomen -- Gastrointestinal bleeding -- Burns and inhalational injury. |
| *Subjects* | Critical care medicine--Handbooks, manuals, etc.<br>Surgical intensive care--Handbooks, manuals, etc.<br>Critical Care--methods.<br>Emergencies.<br>Intensive Care--methods. |
| *Notes* | Includes bibliographical references and index. |

**Critical care nursing: learning from practice**

| | |
|---|---|
| *LCCN* | 2010040962 |
| *Type of material* | Book |
| *Main title* | Critical care nursing: learning from practice / edited by Suzanne Bench and Kate Brown. |
| *Published/Created* | Chichester, West Sussex, UK: Wiley-Blackwell, 2011. |
| *Description* | x, 290 p.: ill.; 25 cm. |
| *ISBN* | 9781405169950 (pbk.: alk. paper) |
| *LC classification* | RT120.I5 C763 2011 |
| *Related names* | Bench, Suzanne.<br>Brown, Kate, MSc. |
| *Contents* | The patient with acute lung injury / Julie Hamilton -- The patient who requiring complex weaning from mechanical ventilation / Cheryl Crocker -- The patient with a fever / Kate Brown -- The patient with severe sepsis / Suzanne Bench -- The patient following cardiac surgery / Maureen Coombs -- The patient with severe upper gastrointestinal bleeding due to oesophageal varices / Suzanne Sargent -- The patient |

with altered blood sugar / Danielle Fullwood -- The patient with increased abdominal pressure / Suzanne Bench -- The patient with acute kidney injury / Annette Davies and Suzanne Bench -- The patient in acute pain / Tina Moore -- The patient requiring sedation / Sinead Mehigan -- The patient with raised intracranial pressure / Deborah Slade -- The patient with confusion / Deborah Slade and Kate Brown -- The patient with seizures / Claire Merriman -- The patient following poisoning / Sue Whaley -- The patient requiring long term care / Ruth Cork.

| | |
|---|---|
| *Subjects* | Intensive care nursing--Case studies.<br>Critical Illness--nursing--Case Reports.<br>Critical Care--methods--Case Reports.<br>Critical Care--organization and administration--Case Reports. |
| *Notes* | Includes bibliographical references and index. |

**Cystatins: protease inhibitors, biomarkers, and immunomodulators**

| | |
|---|---|
| *LCCN* | 2010051528 |
| *Type of material* | Book |
| *Main title* | Cystatins: protease inhibitors, biomarkers, and immunomodulators / John B. Cohen and Linda P. Ryseck, editors. |
| *Published/Created* | New York: Nova Science, c2011. |
| *Description* | xiii, 269 p.: ill.; 26 cm. |
| *ISBN* | 9781612093437 (hardcover)<br>1612093434 (hardcover) |
| *LC classification* | QP609.C94 C94 2011 |
| *Related names* | Cohen, John B.<br>Ryseck, Linda P. |
| *Contents* | Cystatins: the multifaceted protease inhibitors / Medha Priyadarshini, Bilqees Bano -- Anti-trypanosomatid properties of cystatin superfamily: implications on parasite development and virulence / André Luis Souza dos Santos, Claudia Masini d'Avila-Levy, Marta Helena Branquinha -- Calpain-like proteins in trypanosomatids: effects of calpain inhibitors on the parasites' physiology and motivations for their possible |

| | |
|---|---|
| | application as chemotherapeutic agents / André Luis Souza dos Santos, Claudia Masini d'Avila-Levy, Marta Helena Branquinha -- Cystatin C in acute coronary syndromes: the investigation should go on / S. Ferraro ... [et al.] -- Cystatin C and acute kidney injury / M. Guillouet ... [et al.] -- Cystatin C, atherosclerosis and lipid-lowering therapy by statins / T.A. Korolenko ... [et al.] -- Effect of temperature, wavelength, PH, ion pair reagents and organic modifiers' concentration on the elution of cystatin C. stability of mobile phase / Othman Ibrahem Yousef Al-Musaimi, Manar Khalid Fayyad, Adel Khalil Mishal -- Role of cystatin C in the neurodegenerative process and its possible use as a nervous system biomarker / Enrique Juarez Aguilar, Fabio Garcia-Garcia, Maria Teresa Croda Todd -- Cystatin C as a GFR marker in renal transplantation: promises and challenges / Ingrid Masson ... [et al.] -- Cystatin C in HIV patients: not just another GFR marker / Amandine Brunon, Chrisophe Mariat, Pierre Delanaye -- Salivary cystatins and periodontal diseases: a protective role? / Marcia Regina Soares, Lorena Da Ras Gonsalves -- Cystatins / Eri S. Srivatsan. |
| *Subjects* | Cystatins.<br>Cysteine proteinases--Inhibitors.<br>Cystatins. |
| *Notes* | Includes bibliographical references and index. |
| *Series* | Protein science and engineering<br>Protein science and engineering. |

**Dietitian's handbook of enteral and parenteral nutrition**

| | |
|---|---|
| *LCCN* | 2010046076 |
| *Type of material* | Book |
| *Main title* | Dietitian's handbook of enteral and parenteral nutrition / edited by Annalynn Skipper. |
| *Edition* | 3rd ed. |
| *Published/Created* | Sudbury, MA: Jones and Bartlett Learning, c2012. |
| *Description* | xx, 351 p.: ill.; 27 cm. |
| *ISBN* | 9780763742904 |

| | |
|---|---|
| | 0763742902 |
| *LC classification* | RM225 .D54 2012 |
| *Portion of title* | Enteral and parenteral nutrition |
| *Related names* | Skipper, Annalynn. |
| *Contents* | Nutrition support practice in context -- Nutrition screening and assessment -- Nutrition support: indication and efficacy -- An ethics primer -- Indirect calorimetry -- Macronutrient requirements -- Water and micronutrients -- Nutrition needs of neonates -- Unique nutrient needs of the geriatric patient -- Acute and chronic pancreatitis -- Nutrition support in liver disease -- Acute kidney injury -- Solid organ transplant -- HIV and cancer -- Burns -- Surgery and wound healing -- Trauma -- Obesity in critical illness -- Enteral feeding -- Parenteral nutrition -- Nutrition support in the acute care environment. |
| *Subjects* | Enteral feeding--Handbooks, manuals, etc.<br>Parenteral feeding--Handbooks, manuals, etc.<br>Enteral Nutrition.<br>Nutritional Physiological Phenomena.<br>Parenteral Nutrition. |
| *Notes* | Includes bibliographical references and index. |

**Emergency department critical care**

| | |
|---|---|
| *LCCN* | 2012039791 |
| *Type of material* | Book |
| *Main title* | Emergency department critical care / edited by Donald M. Yealy, Clifton W. Callaway. |
| *Published/Created* | Oxford: Oxford University Press, c2013. |
| *Description* | xv, 208 p.: ill.; 21 cm. |
| *ISBN* | 9780199779123 (pbk: alk. paper)<br>9780199976355 (alk. paper)<br>9780199976362 (alk. paper) |
| *LC classification* | RC86.7 .E5652 2013 |
| *Related names* | Yealy, Donald M.<br>Callaway, Clifton W. |
| *Contents* | Approach to undifferentiated organ failure/shock ("blue or bad") / Lily Emlet -- Sepsis and shock with infection / Alan Jones -- Respiratory failure (including |

| | |
|---|---|
| | parenchymal, vascular, and central causes) / Dave Gaieski -- Acute heart failure / Frank Peacock -- Acute MI, acute coronary syndromes, dysrhythmias, pacemakers, and aicds / Robert O'Connor -- Acute kidney injury in the emergency department / John Kellum -- Coma and altered mental status / J. Stephen Huff -- Post-cardiac arrest care / Steve Trecziak -- Intracranial hemorrhage and acute ischemic stroke / Ed Jauch -- Management of the critically poisoned patient / Eric Lavonas -- Multisystem trauma and burns / Raquel Forsythe -- Massive bleeding including GI / Charles Wira -- Procedural analgesia and sedation: moderate and deep / John Burton -- Monitoring technology: invasive and non-invasive / Bryant Nguyen -- Airway management / Henry Wang -- Ultrasound for shock / Robert Hyde -- Blood product and procoagulant therapies / Ed Sloan. |
| *Subjects* | Critical Care--methods.<br>Critical Illness--therapy.<br>Emergency Service, Hospital.<br>Emergency Treatment--methods. |
| *Notes* | Includes bibliographical references and index. |
| *Series* | Pittsburgh critical care medicine series<br>Pittsburgh critical care medicine. |

**Essentials of chronic kidney disease**

| | |
|---|---|
| *LCCN* | 2015936099 |
| *Type of material* | Book |
| *Main title* | Essentials of chronic kidney disease / Stephen Z. Fadem, MD, editor. |
| *Published/Created* | New York: Nova Science, c2015. |
| *Description* | xx, 389 p.: col. ill.; 25 cm. |
| *ISBN* | 163482542X<br>9781634825429 |
| *LC classification* | RC918.R4 E72 2015 |
| *Related names* | Fadem, Stephen Z. |
| *Contents* | Defining, classifying and staging chronic kidney disease / Morgan Grams, MD -- Selecting the right estimated glomerular filtration rate / Andrew S. Leevy, |

MD -- Reversing the reversible / Stephen Z. Fadem, MD -- Preventing chronic kidney disease: an overview / Stephen Z. Fadem, MD -- Imaging in chronic kidney disease / Barry Toombs, MD -- Screening for chronic kidney disease: critical analysis / Richard J. Glassock, MD -- Using guidelines in the approach to the chronic kidney disease patient / Garabed Eknoyan, MD -- Acute kidney injury: classification and prognosis / Biruh Workeneh, MD -- Nutritional therapy for patients with chronic kidney disease / William E. Mitch, MD -- Medications to avoid in chronic kidney disease / Sarah McDaniel, PharmD and William M. Bennett, MD -- The role of blood pressure control and anti-hypertensive therapy in preventing kidney disease progression / Jordana B. Cohen, MD and Raymond R. Townsend, MD -- The approach to glomerular disease in chronic kidney disease / Wooin Ahn, MD, Andrew Bomback, MD and Gerald Appel, MD -- The approach to hematuria in chronic kidney disease / Woon Ahn, MD, Andrew Bomback, MD and Gerald Appel, MD -- Diabetic nephropathy: current clinical challenges / Mark E. Williams, MD and Sylvia E. Rosas, MD -- Focal segmental glomerulosclerosis and collapsing glomerulopathy syndromes / Jeffrey B. Knopp, MD -- APOL 1 kidney disease / Jeffrey B. Kopp, MD and Cheryl A. Winkler, PhD -- Uric acid and chronic kidney disease / Anuradha Wadhwa, MD and Richard J. Johnson, MD -- Other causes of chronic kidney disease / Anjay Rastogi, MD, PhD, and Mehdi Momen, MD -- When to refer the chronic kidney disease patient to the nephrologist / Willaim H. Herman, MD, MPH, and Richard Hellman, MD -- Transitions of care in a complex patient population: the case of chronic kidney disease / Todd F. Griffith, MD and J. Edward Hartle II, MD -- Disease management strategies in chronic kidney disease / Robert J. Kossmann, MD -- Approach to the psychological aspects of chronic kidney disease / Emily Steinberg Fadem, MD -- Whether to initiate dialysis therapy in

| | |
|---|---|
| | geriatric patients with advanced chronic kidney disease / Eli A. Friedman, MD -- Cardiovascular disease in chronic kidney disease / Peter A. McCullough, MD -- Anemia in chronic kidney disease / Muzzaffar Hussain, MD and Michael J. Germain, MD -- Metabolic acidosis and management with dietary alkali / Donald E. Wesson, MD -- The low serum albumin in chronic kidney disease / Allon N. Friedman, MD -- Chronic kidney disease - mineral bone disorder / Ruth L. Wintz, MD and Antonio Duran, MD -- Keeping patients employed / Robert Provenzano, MD -- Assessing and preparing the patient for future ESRD modalities / Martin J. Schreiber, MD and Thomas A. Golper, MD -- Prognostication tools as a guide to appropriate integration of palliative care into chronic kidney disease treatment plans / Jennifer S. Scherer, MD and Michael J. Germain, MD -- When renal replacement therapy may not be the best option / Rebecca Schmidt, MD -- Assessing the chronic kidney disease patient's vessels for hemodialysis vascular access / Vo D. Nguyen, MD -- Peritoneal dialysis / John Burkart, MD -- Home hemodialysis / Robert S. Lockridge Jr., MD -- In-center nocturnal hemodialysis / Rachel Fissel, MD -- Staff assisted in-center hemodialysis / Douglas S. Johnson, MD, Toros Kapoian, MD, and Klemens B. Meyer, MD -- Preemptive kidney transplantation / Horacio E. Adrogue, MD. |
| *Subjects* | Chronic renal failure.<br>Kidneys--Diseases.<br>Chronic renal failure.<br>Kidneys--Diseases. |
| *Notes* | Includes bibliographical references and index. |
| *Series* | Renal, metabolic and urologic disorders<br>Renal, metabolic and urologic disorders. |

**Fluid overload: diagnosis and management**

| | |
|---|---|
| *LCCN* | 2010007012 |
| *Type of material* | Book |

| | |
|---|---|
| *Main title* | Fluid overload: diagnosis and management / volume editors, Claudio Ronco ... [et al.]. |
| *Published/Created* | Basel [Switzerland]; New York: Karger, c2010. |
| *Description* | viii, 243 p.: ill.; 25 cm. |
| *ISBN* | 9783805594165 (hc: alk. paper)<br>380559416X |
| *LC classification* | RC630 .F585 2010 |
| *Related names* | Ronco, C. (Claudio), 1951- |
| *Contents* | Heart failure: pathophysiology and clinical picture / Palazzuoli, A., Nuti, R. -- Heart failure classifications: guidelines / Jankowska, E.A., Ponikowski, P. -- Acute kidney injury: classification and staging / Cruz, D.N. ... [et al.] -- Cardiorenal syndromes: definition and classification / Ronco, C. -- Oliguria and fluid overload / Rimmelâe, T., Kellum, J.A. -- Pathophysiology of fluid retention in heart failure / Chaney, E., Shaw, A. -- Fluid overload as a biomarker of heart failure and acute kidney injury / Bagshaw, S.M., Cruz, D.N. -- Fluid balance issues in the critically ill patient / Bouchard, J., Mehta, R.L. -- Prerenal azotemia in congestive heart failure / Macedo, E., Mehta, R. -- Use of biomarkers in evaluation of patients with heart failure / Slavin, L., Daniels, L.B., Maisel, A.S. -- Oliguria, creatinine and other biomarkers of acute kidney injury / Ronco, C. ... [et al.] -- Current techniques of fluid status assessment / Peacock, W.F., Soto, K.M. -- Bioelectric impedance measurement for fluid status assessment / Piccoli, A. - Diuretic therapy in fluid-overloaded and heart failure patients / Bellomo, R., Prowle, J.R., Echeverri, J.E. -- Pharmacological therapy of cardiorenal syndromes and heart failure / House, A.A. -- Extracorporeal fluid removal in heart failure patients / Costanzo, M.R., Agostoni, P., Marenzi, G. -- Technical aspects of extracorporeal ultrafiltration: mechanisms, monitoring, and dedicated technology / Nalesso, F., Garzotto, F., Ronco, C. -- Use of brain natriuretic peptide and bioimpedance to guide therapy in heart failure patients / Valle, R., Aspromonte, N. -- Fluid management in |

| | |
|---|---|
| | pediatric intensive care / Favia, I. ... [et al.] -- Fluid assessment and management in the emergency department / Di Somma, S. ... [et al.]. |
| *Subjects* | Body fluid disorders.<br>Congestive heart failure--Complications.<br>Heart Failure.<br>Body Fluids.<br>Kidney Failure, Acute.<br>Oliguria.<br>Water-Electrolyte Balance. |
| *Notes* | Includes bibliographical references and indexes. |
| *Series* | Contributions to nephrology, 0302-5144; v. 164<br>Contributions to nephrology; v. 164. |

**Geriatric emergencies**

| | |
|---|---|
| *LCCN* | 2014034303 |
| *Type of material* | Book |
| *Personal name* | Murdoch, Iona, 1984- , author. |
| *Main title* | Geriatric emergencies / Iona Murdoch, Sarah Turpin, Bree Johnston, Alasdair MacLullich, Eve Losman. |
| *Published/Produced* | Chichester, West Sussex; Ames, Iowa: John Wiley and Sons Inc., 2015. |
| *ISBN* | 9781118655573 (cloth) |
| *LC classification* | RC86.7 |
| *Related names* | Turpin, Sarah, 1985- , author.<br>Johnston, Bree, author.<br>MacLullich, Alasdair, author.<br>Losman, Eve, author. |
| *Contents* | Introduction to geriatric emergency medicine -- Essentials of assessment and management in geriatric emergency medicine -- Special skills in geriatric emergency medicine -- Vulnerable adults and elder abuse -- Chest pain and atrial fibrillation -- Dyspnoea -- Infection and sepsis -- Falls and immobility -- Syncope -- Dizziness -- Major trauma -- Fractures and back pain -- Skin trauma -- Head injury -- Abdominal emergencies -- Diabetic and environmental emergencies -- Acute kidney injury and metabolic emergencies -- Delirium -- Stroke and transient |

| | |
|---|---|
| | ischaemic attack. |
| *Subjects* | Aged. |
| | Emergencies. |
| | Emergency Treatment--methods. |
| *Notes* | Includes bibliographical references and index. |
| *Additional formats* | Online version: Murdoch, Iona, 1984- , author. Geriatric emergencies Chichester, West Sussex; Ames, Iowa: John Wiley and Sons Inc., 2015 9781118655665 (DLC) 2014034943 |

**Handbook of common problems in clinical nephrology**

| | |
|---|---|
| *LCCN* | 2009048912 |
| *Type of material* | Book |
| *Personal name* | Thorp, Micah L. |
| *Main title* | Handbook of common problems in clinical nephrology / Micah L. Thorp. |
| *Published/Created* | New York: Nova Science Publishers, c2010. |
| *Description* | 162 p.: ill.; 23 cm. |
| *ISBN* | 9781608768288 (pbk.) |
| | 1608768287 (pbk.) |
| *LC classification* | RC903 .T48 2010 |
| *Contents* | Elevated serum creatinine -- Evaluation of proteinuria -- Evaluation of hematuria -- Chronic kidney disease management -- Acute kidney injury -- Electrolyte disorders -- Acid/base disorders -- Hypertension -- Pregnancy and the kidney -- Nephrolithiasis -- Renal replacement therapies. |
| *Subjects* | Kidneys--Diseases--Handbooks, manuals, etc. |
| | Nephrology--Handbooks, manuals, etc. |
| | Kidney Diseases--diagnosis--Handbooks. |
| | Kidney Diseases--therapy--Handbooks. |
| *Notes* | Includes bibliographical references and index. |
| *Series* | Nephrology research and clinical developments series |

**Harrison's nephrology and acid-base disorders**

| | |
|---|---|
| *LCCN* | 2012039926 |
| *Type of material* | Book |
| *Main title* | Harrison's nephrology and acid-base disorders / editors, J. Larry Jameson, Joseph Loscalzo. |

| | |
|---|---|
| *Edition* | 2nd ed. |
| *Published/Created* | New York: McGraw-Hill Medical, c2013. |
| *Description* | ix, 326 p.: ill. (some col.); 28 cm. |
| *ISBN* | 9780071814966 (pbk.: alk. paper)<br>0071814965 (pbk.: alk. paper) |
| *LC classification* | RC902.A3 H37 2013 |
| *Variant title* | Nephrology and acid-base disorders |
| *Related titles* | Harrison's principles of internal medicine. |
| *Related names* | Jameson, J. Larry.<br>Loscalzo, Joseph.<br>Harrison, Tinsley Randolph, 1900-1978. |
| *Contents* | Cellular and molecular biology of the kidney / Alfred L. George Jr., Eric G. Neilson -- Adaptation of the kidney to renal injury / Raymond C. Harris, Eric G. Neilson -- Azotemia and urinary abnormalities / Julie Lin, Bradley M. Denker -- Atlas of urinary sediments and renal biopsies / Agnes B. Fogo, Eric G. Neilson -- Acidosis and alkalosis / Thomas D. Dubose Jr. -- Fluid and electrolyte disturbances / David B. Mount -- Hypercalcemia and hypocalcemia / Sundeep Khosla -- Hyperuricemia and gout / Christopher M. Burns ... [et al.] -- Nephrolithiasis / John R. Asplin, Fredric L. Coe, Murray J. Favus -- Acute kidney injury / Sushrut S. Waikar, Joseph V. Bonventre -- Chronic kidney disease / Joanne M. Bargman, Karl Skorecki -- Dialysis in the treatment of renal failure / Kathleen D. Liu, Glenn M. Chertow -- Transplantation in the treatment of renal failure / Anil Chandraker, Edgar L. Milford, Mohamed H. Sayegh -- Infections in kidney transplant recipients / Robert Finberg, Joyce Fingeroth -- Glomerular diseases / Julia B. Lewis, Eric G. Neilson -- Polycystic kidney disease and other inherited tubular disorders / David J. Salant, Craig E. Gordon -- Tubulointerstitial diseases of the kidney / Laurence H. Beck, David J. Salant -- Vascular injury to the kidney / Stephen C. Textor, Nelson Leung -- Hypertensive vascular disease / Theodore A. Kotchen -- Urinary tract infections, pyelonephritis, and prostatitis / Barbara W. Trautner, Kalpana Gupta -- |

| | |
|---|---|
| | Urinary tract obstruction / Julian L. Seifter -- Bladder and renal cell carcinomas / Howard I. Scher, Robert J. Motzer. |
| *Subjects* | Nephrology.<br>Kidneys--Diseases.<br>Acid-base imbalances.<br>Kidney Diseases.<br>Acid-Base Imbalance.<br>Kidney--pathology. |
| *Notes* | Compilation of chapters related to kidney function from Harrison's principles of internal medicine. 18th ed. 2012.<br>Includes bibliographical references and index. |

**Introduction to critical care nursing**

| | |
|---|---|
| *LCCN* | 2012008134 |
| *Type of material* | Book |
| *Main title* | Introduction to critical care nursing / [edited by] Mary Lou Sole, Deborah G. Klein, Marthe J. Moseley. |
| *Edition* | 6th ed. |
| *Published/Created* | St. Louis, Mo.: Elsevier/Saunders, c2013. |
| *Description* | xxii, 740 p.: ill.; 28 cm. |
| *ISBN* | 9780323088480 (pbk.: alk. paper) |
| *LC classification* | RT120.I5 I58 2013 |
| *Variant title* | Critical care nursing |
| *Related names* | Sole, Mary Lou.<br>Klein, Deborah G.<br>Moseley, Marthe J. |
| *Contents* | Overview of critical care nursing / Mary Lou Sole -- Patient and family response to the critical care experience / Sandra Knapp, Mary Lou Sole -- Ethical and legal issues in critical care nursing / Jayne Willis, Kathy Black Mary Lou Sole -- End-of-life care in the critical care unit / Douglas Houghton / Mary Lou Sole -- Comfort and sedation / Mamoona Arif-Rahu, Mary Lou Sole -- Nutritional support / Miranda Kelly, Marthe Moseley -- Dysrhythmia interpretation and management / Julie Marcum, Marthe Moseley -- Hemodynamic monitoring / David Allen, Maximino |

| | |
|---|---|
| | Martell, Marthe Moseley -- Ventilatory assistance / Lynelle Pierce, Mary Lou Sole -- Rapid response teams and code management / Deborah Klein -- Shock, sepsis, and multiple organ dysfunction syndrome / Kathleen Hill -- Cardiovascular alterations / Colleen Walsh-Irwin, Marthe Moseley -- Nervous system alterations / Christina Stewart-Amidei, Deborah Klein -- Acute respiratory failure / Maureen Seckel, Mary Lou Sole -- Acute kidney injury / Kathleen Kerber, Deborah Klein -- Hematological and immune disorders / Patricia Wolff, Jill Dickerson, Marthe Moseley -- Gastrointestinal alterations / Katherine (Kaye) Alford, Marthe Moseley -- Endocrine alterations / Christina Stewart-Amidei, Jacqueline LaManna /Marthe Moseley -- Trauma and surgical management / Mary Beth Makic, Deborah Klein -- Burns / Karla Klas, Deborah Klein -- Solid organ transplantation / Linda Ohler, Tracy Evans-Walker, Deborah Klein . |
| *Subjects* | Critical Care. |
| | Nursing Care. |
| *Notes* | Includes bibliographical references and index. |

**Kidney disease management: a practical approach for the non-specialist healthcare practitioner**

| | |
|---|---|
| *LCCN* | 2012032765 |
| *Type of material* | Book |
| *Main title* | Kidney disease management: a practical approach for the non-specialist healthcare practitioner / [edited by] Rachel Lewis, Helen Noble. |
| *Published/Created* | Chichester, West Sussex: John Wiley and Sons, 2013. |
| *ISBN* | 9780470670613 (pbk.) |
| *LC classification* | RC903 |
| *Related names* | Lewis, Rachel, 1965- |
| | Noble, Helen, 1964- |
| *Contents* | Managing chronic conditions: the policy context / Beverley Matthews -- What non-specialists need to know about chronic kidney disease / Graham Woodrow, Jeanette Denning and David Lewis -- A practical approach to managing chronic kidney disease |

| | |
|---|---|
| | in primary care / Hugh Raynor, Raj Pal, and Indaril Dasgupta -- General considerations relating to treatment modalities / Aisha Hussein, Charlie Tomson, Lesley Lappin -- The psychosocial reality of living with chronic kidney disease / Emma Coyne -- Acute kidney injury in hospitalised patients / Keith Harkins, Rachel Lewis, Rachel Hilton -- Reducing the risks associated with surgery and kidney injury / Colin H. Jones and Maggie Higginbotham -- Medication management and chronic kidney disease / Aileen Dunleavy -- Optimising nutrition in people with chronic kidney disease / Helena Jackson and Sally Noble -- Supportive and palliative care / Sheila Johnston and Helen Noble. |
| *Subjects* | Kidney Diseases.<br>Chronic Disease--therapy.<br>Renal Insufficiency, Chronic. |
| *Notes* | Includes bibliographical references and index. |

**Manual of nephrology**

| | |
|---|---|
| *LCCN* | 2014008807 |
| *Type of material* | Book |
| *Main title* | Manual of nephrology / edited by Robert W. Schrier, MD, Professor Emeritus, Division of Renal Disease and Hypertension, University of Colorado Health Sciences Center, Aurora, Colorado. |
| *Edition* | Eighth edition. |
| *Published/Produced* | Philadelphia: Wolters Kluwer Health, [2015] ©2015 |
| *Description* | x, 443 pages: illustrations; 21 cm. |
| *Links* | Table of contents only http://www.loc.gov/catdir/enhancements/fy1408/2014008807-t.html<br>Publisher description http://www.loc.gov/catdir/enhancements/fy1408/2014008807-d.html |
| *ISBN* | 9781451192957 (pbk.)<br>1451192959 (pbk.) |
| *LC classification* | RC903 .M194 2015 |
| *Related names* | Schrier, Robert W., editor. |
| *Contents* | The edematous patient: cardiac failure, cirrhosis, and |

| | |
|---|---|
| | nephrotic syndrome / Robert W. Schrier and David H. Ellison -- The patient with hyponatremia or hypernatremia / Robert W. Schrier and Tomas Berl -- The patient with hypokalemia or hyperkalemia / Jie Tang and Stuart L. Linas -- The patient with an acid-base disorder / William D. Kaehny -- The patient with disorders of serum calcium and phosphorus / Jeffrey G. Penfield and Robert F. Reilly -- The patient with kidney stones / Robert F. Reilly -- The patient with urinary tract infection / Jessica B. Kendrick, L. Barth Reller, and Marilyn E. Levi -- The patient with hematuria, proteinuria, or both, and abnormal findings on urinary microscopy / Godela M. Brosnahan -- The patient with glomerular disease or vasculitis / Sarah E. Panzer and Joshua M. Thurman -- The patient with acute kidney injury / Sarah Faubel and Charles L. Edelstein -- The patient with chronic kidney disease / Michel Chonchol and Jessica B. Kendrick -- The patient receiving chronic renal replacement with dialysis / Seth Ferguson and Isaac Teitelbaum -- The patient with a kidney transplant / James Cooper, Lawrence Chan, and Alexander Wiseman -- The patient with kidney disease and hypertension in pregnancy / Phyllis August, Diana I. Jalal, and Judy Blaine -- The patient with hypertension / Seth Ferguson, Charles R. Nolan, and Robert W. Schrier -- Practical guidelines for drug dosing in patients with impaired kidney function / Ali Olyaei and William M. Bennett. |
| *Subjects* | Kidney Diseases--diagnosis--Handbooks.<br>Kidney Diseases--therapy--Handbooks.<br>Metabolic Diseases--diagnosis--Handbooks.<br>Metabolic Diseases--therapy--Handbooks. |
| *Notes* | Includes bibliographical references and index. |

**Medical nutrition therapy: a case study approach**

| | |
|---|---|
| *LCCN* | 2013931079 |
| *Type of material* | Book |
| *Personal name* | Nahikian-Nelms, Marcia, author. |

| | |
|---|---|
| *Main title* | Medical nutrition therapy: a case study approach / Marcia Nahikian Nelms, PhD, RD, LD, CNSC, Ohio State University; Sara Long Roth, PhD, RD, LD, Southern Illinois University. |
| *Edition* | Fourth edition. |
| *Published/Produced* | Stamford, Connecticut: Cengage Learning, [2014] |
| *Description* | xx, 436 p.; 28 cm. |
| *ISBN* | 9781133593157 (pbk.)<br>1133593151 (pbk.) |
| *LC classification* | RM216 .N246 2014 |
| *Related names* | Roth, Sara Long. |
| *Contents* | Pediatric Weight Management -- Bariatric Surgery for Morbid Obesity -- Malnutrition Associated with Chronic Disease -- Hypertension and Cardiovascular Disease -- Myocardial Infarction -- Heart Failure with Resulting Cardiac Cachexia -- Gastroesophegal Reflux Disease -- Ulcer Disease: Medical and Surgical Treatment -- Celiac Disease -- Irritable Bowel Syndrome -- Inflammatory Bowel Disease: Crohn's Disease -- Cirrhosis of the Liver -- Acute Pancreatitis -- Pediatric Type 1 Diabetes Mellitus -- Type 1 Diabetes Mellitus in the Adult -- Type 2 Diabetes Mellitus--Pediatric Obesity -- Adult Type 2 Diabetes Mellitus: Transition to Insulin -- Chronic Kidney Disease (CKD) Treated with Dialysis -- Chronic Kidney Disease: Peritoneal Dialysis -- Acute Kidney Injury (AKI) -- Anemia in Pregnancy -- Folate and Vitamin B12 Deficiencies -- Ischemic Stroke -- Progressive Neurological Disease: Parkinson's Disease -- Alzheimer's Disease -- Chronic Obstructive Pulmonary Disease -- COPD with Respiratory Failure -- Pediatric Traumatic Brain Injury: Metabolic Stress with Nutrition Support -- Metabolic Stress and Trauma: Open Abdomen -- Nutrition Support for Burn Injury -- Nutrition Support in Sepsis and Morbid Obesity -- Acute Lymphoblastic Leukemia Treated with Hematopoietic Cell Transplantation -- Esophageal Cancer Treated with Surgery and Radiation -- AIDS. |

| | |
|---|---|
| *Subjects* | Diet therapy--Case studies.<br>Diet Therapy--Case Reports.<br>Nutritional Physiological Phenomena--Case Reports.<br>Diet therapy. |
| *Form/Genre* | Case studies. |
| *Notes* | Includes bibliographical references and index. |

**Medical-surgical nursing: assessment and management of clinical problems**

| | |
|---|---|
| *LCCN* | 2010028656 |
| *Type of material* | Book |
| *Main title* | Medical-surgical nursing: assessment and management of clinical problems / Sharon L. Lewis ... [et al.]. |
| *Edition* | 8th ed. |
| *Published/Created* | St. Louis, Mo.: Elsevier/Mosby, c2011. |
| *Description* | 2 v.: ill. (chiefly col.); 29 cm. + 1 DVD-ROM (4 3/4 in.) |
| *ISBN* | 9780323065801 (single v.: hard cover: alk. paper)<br>0323065805 (single v.: hard cover: alk. paper)<br>9780323065818 (two-v. set: hard cover: alk. paper)<br>0323065813 (two-v. set: hard cover: alk. paper)<br>9996080900 (v.1)<br>9789996080906 (v.1)<br>9996080846 (v.2)<br>9789996080845 (v.2) |
| *LC classification* | RT41 .M488 2011 |
| *Related names* | Lewis, Sharon Mantik. |
| *Contents* | V. 1 -- Contemporary nursing practice -- Health disparities and culturally competent care -- Health history and physical examination -- Patient and caregiver teaching -- Chronic illness and older adults -- Community-based nursing and home care -- Complementary and alternative therapies -- Stress and stress management -- Sleep and sleep disorders -- Pain -- Palliative care at end of life -- Addictive behaviors -- Inflammation and wound healing -- Genetics, altered immune responses, and transplantation -- Infection and human immunodeficiency virus infection -- Cancer -- Fluid, electrolyte, and acid-base imbalances -- |

Preoperative care -- Intraoperative care -- Postoperative care -- Visual and auditory systems -- Visual and auditory problems -- Integumentary system -- Burns -- Respiratory system -- Upper respiratory problems -- Lower respiratory problems -- Obstructive pulmonary diseases -- Hematologic system -- Hematologic problems -- Cardiovascular system -- Hypertension -- Coronary artery disease and acute coronary syndrome -- Heart failure -- Dysrhythmias -- Inflammatory and structural heart disorders -- Vascular disorders.
V. 2 -- Gastrointestinal system -- Nutritional problems -- Obesity -- Upper gastrointestinal problems -- Lower gastrointestinal problems -- Liver, pancreas, and biliary tract problems -- Urinary system -- Renal and urologic problems -- Acute kidney injury and chronic kidney disease -- Endocrine system -- Diabetes mellitus -- Endocrine problems -- Reproductive system -- Breast disorders -- Sexually transmitted diseases -- Female reproductive problems -- Male reproductive problems -- Nervous system -- Acute intracranial problems -- Stroke -- Chronic neurologic problems -- Alzheimer's disease, dementia, and delirium -- Peripheral nerve and spinal cord problems -- Musculoskeletal system -- Musculoskeletal trauma and orthopedic surgery -- Musculoskeletal problems -- Arthritis and connective tissue diseases -- Critical care -- Shock, systemic inflammatory response syndrome, and multiple organ dysfunction syndrome -- Respiratory failure and acute respiratory distress syndrome -- Emergency, terrorism, and disaster nursing -- Appendixes A: Cardiopulmonary resuscitation and basic life support for health care providers -- Appendixes B: Nursing diagnoses -- Appendixes C: Laboratory references intervals.

*Subjects* Nursing.
Surgical nursing.
Nursing Care.
Nursing Assessment.

| | |
|---|---|
| | Perioperative Nursing. |
| *Notes* | Includes bibliographical references and index. |
| *Computer file info* | System requirements: Windows XP SP2, Vista or 32-bit Windows 7 operating system. Intel Pentium 4 processor /1 GHz or greater; 65 MB available hard drive space; 512 MB RAM. MAC OS 10.4 x 10.6x operating system; Intel-based processor or Power PC G4/G5 (867 MHz or higher); 65 MB available hard drive space. |

**Medical-surgical nursing: assessment and management of clinical problems**

| | |
|---|---|
| *LCCN* | 2013036087 |
| *Type of material* | Book |
| *Personal name* | Lewis, Sharon Mantik, author. |
| *Main title* | Medical-surgical nursing: assessment and management of clinical problems / Sharon L. Lewis, RN, PhD, FAAN, Professor Emerita, University of New Mexico, Albuquerque, New Mexico, Former Castella Distinguished Professor, School of Nursing, University of Texas Health Science Center at San Antonio, San Antonio, texas, Developer and Consultant, Stress Busting Program for Family Caregivers, Shannon Ruff Dirksen, RN, PhD, FAAN, Associate Professor, College of Nursing and Health Innovation, Arizona State University, Phoenix, Arizona, Margaret McLean Heitkemper, RN, PhD, FAAN, Professor and Chairperson, Biobehavioral Nursing and Health Systems, Elizabeth Sterling Soule Endowed Chair in Nursing, School of Nursing, Adjunct Professor, Division of Gastroenterology, School of Medicine, University of Washington, Seattle, Washington, Linda Bucher, RN, PhD, CEN, CNE, Emerita Professor, School of Nursing, University of Delaware, Newark, Delaware, Consultant/Mentor, W. Cary Edwards School of Nursing, thomas Edison state College, Trenton, New Jersey, Per Diem Staff Nurse, Emergency Department, Virtua Memorial Hospital, Mt. Holly, New Jersey; special editor, Mariann M. |

| | |
|---|---|
| | Harding, RN, PhD, CNE, Associate Professor of Nursing, Kent State University at Tuscarawas, New Philadelphia, Ohio. |
| *Edition* | Ninth edition. |
| *Published/Produced* | St. Louis, Missouri: Elsevier/Mosby, [2014] |
| *Description* | 2 volumes (xxxi, 1708 pages, 82 variously numbered pages): color illustrations; 28 cm |
| *ISBN* | 9780323100892 (two volume set, pbk.: alk. paper)<br>0323100899 (two volume set, pbk.: alk. paper)<br>9780323086783 (single volume, hardcover: alk. paper)<br>0323086780 (single volume, hardcover: alk. paper) |
| *LC classification* | RT41 .M488 2014 |
| *Related names* | Dirksen, Shannon Ruff, author.<br>Heitkemper, Margaret M. (Margaret McLean), author.<br>Bucher, Linda, author.<br>Harding, Mariann, editor. |
| *Contents* | Professional nursing practice -- Health disparities and culturally competent care -- Health history and physical examination -- Patient and caregiver teaching -- Chronic illness and older adults -- Complementary and alternative therapies -- Stress and stress management -- Sleep and sleep disorders -- Pain -- Palliative care at end of life -- Substance abuse -- Pathophysiologic mechanisms of disease -- Inflammation and wound healing -- Genetics and genomics -- Altered immune responses and transplantation -- Infection and human immunodeficiency virus infection -- Cancer -- Fluid, electrolyte, and acid-base imbalances -- Nursing management preoperative care -- Nursing management intraoperative care -- Nursing management postoperative care -- Nursing assessment visual and auditory systems -- Nursing management visual and auditory problems -- Nursing assessment integumentary system -- Nursing management integumentary problems -- Nursing management burns -- Nursing assessment respiratory system -- Nursing management upper respiratory problems -- Nursing management lower respiratory problems -- Nursing |

management obstructive pulmonary diseases -- Nursing assessment hematologic system -- Nursing management hematologic problems -- Nursing assessment cardiovascular system -- Nursing management hypertension -- Nursing management coronary artery disease and acute coronary syndrome -- Nursing management heart failure -- Nursing management dysrhythmias -- Nursing management inflammatory and structural heart disorders -- Nursing management vascular disorders -- Nursing assessment gastrointestinal system -- Nursing management nutritional problems -- Nursing management obesity -- Nursing management upper gastrointestinal problems -- Nursing management lower gastrointestinal problems -- Nursing management liver, pancreas, and biliary tract problems -- Nursing assessment urinary system -- Nursing management renal and urologic problems -- Nursing management acute kidney injury and chronic kidney disease -- Nursing assessment endocrine system -- Nursing management diabetes mellitus -- Nursing management endocrine problems -- Nursing assessment reproductive system -- Nursing management breast disorders -- Nursing management sexually transmitted diseases -- Nursing management female reproductive problems -- Nursing management male reproductive problems -- Nursing assessment nervous system -- Nursing management acute intracranial problems -- Nursing management stroke -- Nursing management chronic neurologic problems -- Nursing management alzheimer's disease and dementia -- Nursing management peripheral nerve and spinal cord problems -- Nursing assessment musculoskeletal system -- Nursing management musculoskeletal trauma and orthopedic surgery -- Nursing management musculoskeletal problems -- Nursing management arthritis and connective tissue diseases -- Nursing management critical care -- Nursing management shock and multiple organ dysfunction syndrome -- Nursing management respiratory failure and acute respiratory distress syndrome -- Nursing management emergency, terrorism, and disaster nursing.

*Subjects* Nursing Care.
Nursing Assessment.
Perioperative Nursing.

*Notes* Preceded by: Medical-surgical nursing: assessment and management of clinical problems / Sharon L. Lewis ... [et al.]. 8th ed. c2011.
Includes bibliographical references and index.

**Nephrology in 30 days**

*LCCN* 2013006954

*Type of material* Book

*Main title* Nephrology in 30 days / Robert F. Reilly, Mark A. Perazella, [editors].

*Edition* 2nd ed.

*Published/Created* New York: McGraw-Hill, c2014.

*Description* xiii, 402 p.: ill. (chiefly col.); 24 cm.

*Links* Contributor biographical information http://www.loc.gov/catdir/enhancements/fy1311/2013006954-b.html
Publisher description http://www.loc.gov/catdir/enhancements/fy1311/2013006954-d.html

*ISBN* 9780071788403 (alk. paper)
0071788409

*LC classification* RC902.A1 N43 2014

*Variant title* Nephrology in thirty days

*Related names* Reilly, Robert F., M.D.
Perazella, Mark A.

*Contents* Introduction / Mark A. Perazella -- Disorders of Na balance / Robert F. Reilly Jr. -- Disorders of water balance: hypo and hypernatremia / Robert F. Reilly Jr. -- Diuretics / Mark A. Perazella and Mandana Rastegar -- Intelligent use of IV fluids / Robert F. Reilly Jr. -- Disorders of potassium homeostasis: hypo and hyperkalemia / Mark A. Perazella and Maddana Rastegar -- Metabolic acidosis / Adam M. Franks and Joseph I. Shapiro -- Metabolic alkalosis / Adam M. Franks and Joseph I. Shapiro -- Respiratory and mixed acid-base disturbances / Adam M. Franks and Joseph I.

| | |
|---|---|
| | Shapiro -- Disorders of calcium homeostasis: hypo and hypercalcemia / Nishank Jain and Robert F. Reilly Jr. -- Disorders of phosphate homeostasis: hypo and hyperphosphatemia / Nishank Jain and Robert F. Reilly Jr. -- Disorders of magnesium homeostasis: hypo and hypermagnesemia / Robert F. Reilly Jr. -- Nephrolithiasis / Robert F. Reilly Jr. -- Urinalysis and urine microscopy / Mark A. Perazella -- Acute kidney injury / Mark A. Perazella and Mandana Rastegar -- Chronic kidney disease / Mark A. Perazella and Edgar Lerma -- Glomerular diseases / Robert F. Reilly Jr. and Mark A. Perazella -- Tubulointerstitial diseases / Mark A. Perazella and Edgar Lerma -- Urinary obstruction / Richard Formica -- Essential hypertension / Sergio S.S. Santos and Aldo Peixoto -- Secondary causes of hypertension / Sergio S.S. Santos and Aldo Peixoto -- Infection of the urinary tract / Richard Formica. |
| *Subjects* | Kidney Diseases.<br>Metabolic Diseases. |
| *Notes* | Includes bibliographical references and index. |

**Nursing acutely ill adults**

| | |
|---|---|
| *LCCN* | 2015004456 |
| *Type of material* | Book |
| *Personal name* | Woodrow, Philip, 1957- , author. |
| *Main title* | Nursing acutely ill adults / written by Philip Woodrow. |
| *Published/Produced* | Milton Park, Abingdon, Oxon; New York, NY: Routledge, 2015. |
| *Description* | xv, 356 pages: illustrations; 25 cm. |
| *ISBN* | 9781138018877 (hbk)<br>9781138018884 (pbk.) |
| *LC classification* | RT120.I5 W65 2015 |
| *Contents* | The deteriorating patient -- Vital signs -- Blood results -- Respiratory failure -- Oxygen therapy -- Airway management -- Intrepleural chest drainage -- Arterial blood gas interpretation -- Non-invasive ventilation -- Perfusion -- Heart failure -- Acute coronary syndromes and recovery from acute heart failure Shock -- Cardiac rhythms -- Haemaglobinopathies -- Vascular access -- |

| | |
|---|---|
| | Neurological deficits -- Psychological needs -- Thermoregulation -- Acute pain management -- End-of-life care -- Tissue donation -- Fluid balance -- Acute kidney injury -- Fluid management -- Gut function failure -- Diabetic emergencies -- Nutrition -- Infection control -- Accountability. |
| *Subjects* | Critical Care Nursing--methods.<br>Critical Illness--nursing.<br>Critical Care--methods. |
| *Notes* | Includes bibliographical references and index. |

**Nutrition in kidney disease**

| | |
|---|---|
| *LCCN* | 2013956355 |
| *Type of material* | Book |
| *Main title* | Nutrition in kidney disease / Laura D. Byham-Gray, Jerrilynn D. Burrowes, Glenn M. Chertow, editors. |
| *Edition* | 2nd ed. |
| *Published/Created* | New York: Humana, c2014. |
| *Description* | xxxv, 478 p.: ill., ports.; 26 cm. |
| *ISBN* | 9781627036849 (alk. paper)<br>1627036849 (alk. paper) |
| *LC classification* | RC903 .N876 2014 |
| *Related names* | Byham-Gray, Laura.<br>Burrowes, Jerrilynn D.<br>Chertow, Glenn M. |
| *Contents* | Machine generated contents note: pt. I Foundations for Clinical Practice and Overview -- 1.Kidney Function in Health and Disease / Kishore Kuppasani -- 2.Global Perspective of Kidney Disease / Fredric O. Finkelstein -- 3.Dietary Assessment in Kidney Disease / Linda W. Moore -- 4.Anthropometric Assessment in Kidney Disease / Francis Dumler -- 5.Biochemical Nutritional Assessment in Chronic Kidney Disease / David B. Cockram -- 6.Nutrition Physical Assessment in Chronic Kidney Disease (CKD) / Mary Pat Kelly -- pt. II Chronic Kidney Disease Among Adults -- 7.Hypertension / Kristie J. Lancaster -- 8.Diabetes Mellitus and Chronic Kidney Disease (Stages 1 -- 5) / Arti Sharma Parpia -- 9.Dyslipidemias / Wendy E. |

| | |
|---|---|
| | Ramirez -- 10.Implications and Management of Obesity in Kidney Disease / Allon N. Friedman -- pt. III Kidney Disease in Adults Treated by Renal Replacement Therapies -- 11.Dialysis / Karen Wiesen -- 12.Transplantation / Maureen P. McCarthy -- 13.Protein-Energy Wasting / Kamyar Kalantar-Zadeh -- 14.Acute Kidney Injury / Marcia A. Kalista-Richards -- 15.Bone and Mineral Disorders / Linda McCann -- 16.Physical Activity and Exercise / Patricia Painter -- pt. IV Nutrition in Chronic Kidney Disease Among Special Needs Populations -- 17.Pregnancy / Jean Stover -- 18.Infancy, Childhood, and Adolescence / Bradley A. Warady -- 19.The Aging Adult / Julie Barboza -- 20.Nephrotic Syndrome / George A. Kaysen -- 21.Nephrolithiasis / Julian L. Seifter -- pt. V Additional Nutritional Considerations in Kidney Disease -- 22.Public Policy and Renal Nutrition Practice: Past, Present, and Future / Mary H. Hager -- 23.Dietary Supplements / Diane Rigassio Radler -- 24.Vitamin and Trace Element Needs in Chronic Kidney Disease / Joel D. Kopple -- 25.Issues Affecting Dietary Adherence / Jerrilynn D. Burrowes -- 26.Counseling Approaches / Jerrilynn D. Burrowes -- 27.Outcomes Research / Laura D. Byham-Gray. |
| *Subjects* | Kidneys--Diseases--Nutritional aspects.<br>Kidney Diseases--diet therapy.<br>Chronic Disease--prevention and control.<br>Nutritional Physiological Phenomena. |
| *Notes* | Includes bibliographical references and index. |
| *Series* | Nutrition and health<br>Nutrition and health (Totowa, N.J.) |

**Nutritional management of hospitalized small animals**

| | |
|---|---|
| *LCCN* | 2015007221 |
| *Type of material* | Book |
| *Main title* | Nutritional management of hospitalized small animals / edited by Daniel L. Chan. |
| *Published/Produced* | Chichester, West Sussex; Ames, Iowa: John Wiley and Sons Inc., 2015. |

| | |
|---|---|
| *ISBN* | 9781444336474 (cloth) |
| *LC classification* | SF95 .N888 2015 |
| *Related names* | Chan, Daniel L., 1973- , editor. |
| *Contents* | Nutritional assessment / Kathryn E. Michel -- Estimating energy requirements / Daniel L. Chan -- Routes of nutritional support / Sally Perea -- Nasoesophageal feeding tubes / Isuru Gajanayake -- Esophagostomy feeding tubes / Laura Eirmann -- Gastrostomy feeding tubes / Isuru Gajanayake, Daniel L. Chan -- Esophagostomy feeding tubes / Laura Eirmann -- Minimally invasive placement of post-pyloric feeding tubes / Matthew W. Beal -- Tube feeding: diet selection and preparation / Iveta Becvarova -- Intravenous access for parenteral nutrition / Sophie Adamantos -- Parenteral nutrition / Daniel L. Chan and Lisa M. Freeman -- Pathophysiology and clinical approach to malnutrition / Jason W. Gagne and Joseph J. Wakshlag -- Appetite stimulants / Lisa P. Weeth -- Adverse food reactions / Cecilia Villaverde and Marta Hervera -- Nutritional management of short bowel syndrome / Daniel L. Chan -- Refeeding syndrome / Daniel L. Chan -- Feeding patients with gastrointestinal motility disorders / Karin Allenspach and Daniel L. Chan -- Immune modulating nutrients / Daniel L. Chan -- Nutritional management of superficial necrolytic dermatitis / Andrea V. Volk and Ross Bond -- Nutritional support in acute kidney injury / Denise A. Elliott -- Nutritional support in hepatic failure / Renee M. Streeter and Joseph J. Wakshlag -- Nutritional management of the septic patient / Daniel L. Chan -- Nutritional support during acute pancreatitis / Kristine B. Jensen and Daniel L. Chan -- Nutritional support in the mechanically ventilated small animal patient / Daniel L. Chan -- Nutritional support in exotic pet species / Jeleen A. Briscoe, La'Toya Latney, and Cailin R. Heinze. |
| *Subjects* | Animal nutrition.<br>Veterinary nursing. |

| | |
|---|---|
| | Animal feeding.<br>Veterinary diet therapy.<br>Animal Nutritional Physiological Phenomena.<br>Nutritional Support--veterinary.<br>Nutritional Requirements.<br>Nutritional Status.<br>Veterinary Medicine--methods. |
| *Notes* | Includes bibliographical references and index. |
| *Additional formats* | Online version: Nutritional management of hospitalized small animals Chichester, West Sussex; Ames, Iowa: John Wiley and Sons Inc., 2015 9781119052968 (DLC) 2015015939 |

**OSCEs for the final FFICM**

| | |
|---|---|
| *LCCN* | 2016011814 |
| *Type of material* | Book |
| *Personal name* | Nichani, Raj, author. |
| *Main title* | OSCEs for the final FFICM / Raj Nichani, Brendan McGrath. |
| *Published/Produced* | Cambridge; New York: Cambridge University Press, 2016. |
| *ISBN* | 9781107579453 (paperback) |
| *LC classification* | RC86.8 |
| *Related names* | McGrath, Brendan, 1974- , author. |
| *Summary* | "This study guide includes in-depth coverage of past FFICM exam material, and is an invaluable resource for trainees preparing for the OSCE examination in intensive care medicine. A structured layout gives the reader clear and convenient access to a wealth of model questions and answers that can be used for quick-fire practice or more detailed study. The book is divided into four sections covering data interpretation, equipment, ethics and communication, and resuscitation and simulation. Questions have been matched to the curriculum, ensuring accurate and comprehensive revision guidance, and a sample marking scheme is provided to assist with exam preparation. Incorporating recommendations from the FFICM Court of Examiners, additional data analysis, |

images and ECGs are included to build on common areas of potential improvement"--Provided by publisher.

*Contents* Machine generated contents note: Part I. Data Interpretation: 1. Acid base; 2. Methaemoglobin; 3. Infective diarrhoea and toxic megacolon; 4. Major burn; 5. Ruptured hemidiaphragm; 6. Post cardiac arrest; 7. Necrotising fasciitis; 8. ARDS; 9. Stridor; 10. Hyponatraemia; 11. Chest drain in liver; 12. Interpretation of pulmonary function tests; 13. Serotonin syndrome; 14. Propofol infusion syndrome; 15. Guillain-Barre; syndrome; 16. Epidural management; 17. Panton-Valentine leukocidin (PVL) MRSA pneumonia; 18. Surviving (urological) sepsis; 19. Ventilator associated pneumonia; 20. Refeeding syndrome; 21. Acute coronary syndrome and papillary muscle rupture; 22. TTP/HUS; 23. Subarachnoid haemorrhage; 24. Post oesophagectomy anastomotic leak; 25. Pulmonary embolism; 26. Heparin-induced thrombocytopenia; 27. Brainstem death; 28. Tricyclic overdose; 29. Chest pain assessment; 30. Intra abdominal hypertension; 31. Selective decontamination of the digestive tract; 32. Bone marrow transplant; 33. Acute kidney injury; 34. Broncho-pleural fistula; 35. Myasthenia gravis; 36. RV infarct; 37. Rhabdomyolysis; 38. Cerebrovascular accident; 39. Acute leukaemia; 40. Diabetic keto acidosis; 41. Failure to wean; 42. Pleural effusion; 43. ICU follow up clinic anaemia; 44. Acute liver failure; 45. Cirrhosis with upper GI bleeding; 46. Sedation and sedation scoring; 47. Encephalitis, epilepsy and MRI scans; 48. Acute renal failure in a HIV positive man; 49. Digoxin toxicity and cardiac pacing; 50. Acute pancreatitis; 51. Cortisol and thyroxine in the critically ill; 52. TEG and major haemorrhage; 53. Poisoning; 54. ECG interpretation; 55. CXR interpretation; Part II. Equipment: 1. Arterial lines; 2. Tracheostomy weaning and communication; 3. Bronchoscopy; 4. Cooling devices; 5. PA catheter; 6. Naso gastric tubes;

| | |
|---|---|
| | 7. High flow nasal cannula; 8. Cardiac output technologies; 9. Catheter related blood stream infection and vancomycin-resistant enterococcus; 10. Spinal needles; 11. Capnography; 12. Patient transfer; 13. Tracheostomies; 14. Central lines; 15. Haemofiltration; 16. Intra aortic balloon pump; Part III. Ethics and Communication: 1. Anaphylaxis; 2. Pulmonary embolism; 3. Malignant hyperpyrexia; 4. Organ donation; 5. End of life care; 6. Muscular dystrophy; 7. Delirium; 8. Deterioration post discharge; 9. Consent for tracheostomy; 10. Blood transfusion; 11. Alcoholic liver disease; 12. Long QT; Part IV. Resuscitation: Introduction; 1. Displaced airway; 2. Child submersion; 3. Child with seizures; 4. Bleeding trauma with head injury; 5. Asthma; 6. Pregnancy and VF arrest; 7. Chest opening on the ICU; 8. Paediatric sepsis; 9. Tracheostomy emergency; 10. Anaphylaxis. |
| *Subjects* | Critical Care<br>Great Britain |
| *Form/Genre* | Examination Questions |
| *Notes* | Includes bibliographical references and index. |

**Oxford textbook of interventional cardiology**

| | |
|---|---|
| *LCCN* | 2010001498 |
| *Type of material* | Book |
| *Main title* | Oxford textbook of interventional cardiology / edited by Simon Redwood, Nick Curzen and Martyn Thomas. |
| *Published/Created* | New York: Oxford University Press, USA, 2010. |
| *Description* | xv, 734 p.: ill. (some col.); 26 cm. |
| *Links* | Contributor biographical information http://www.loc.gov/catdir/enhancements/fy1102/2010001498-b.html<br>Publisher description http://www.loc.gov/catdir/enhancements/fy1102/2010001498-d.html<br>Table of contents only http://www.loc.gov/catdir/enhancements/fy1102/2010001498-t.html |
| *ISBN* | 9780199569083 (hc)<br>0199569088 |
| *LC classification* | RD598.35.A53 O94 2010 |

*Portion of title* Interventional cardiology

*Related names* Redwood, Simon.
Curzen, Nick.
Thomas, Martyn.

*Summary* "Cardiac catheterization and coronary angiography remain the key tools in the management of patients with coronary heart disease. Interventional cardiology is now routinely performed outside of major cardiac centres, often in small district hospitals. General training in cardiology rarely offers more than the opportunity to assist a more senior operator to perform angioplasty procedures, so a textbook for the non-specialist has become essential reading. Oxford Textbook of Interventional Cardiology is a definitive text spanning the whole spectrum of interventional cardiology procedures, including management of patients with coronary artery disease, one of the leading killers in western society. Written by an expert faculty of international authors, it offers guidance on all aspects of interventional cardiology according to the European curriculum and guidelines for practice, and covers the very latest techniques and devices to provide practical, evidence-based guidance on treating a full range of coronary lesions. The book also covers structural heart disease and new developments in heart valve disease, which were previously in the realm of cardiac surgeons but are now being treated by cardiologists using less invasive methods"--Provided by publisher.

*Contents* Machine generated contents note: -- <strong>Background and basics </strong> -- 1. The epidemiology and pathophysiology of coronary artery disease -- 2. The history of interventional cardiology -- 3. Risk assessment and analysis of outcomes -- 4. Vascular access: femoral versus radial -- 5. Radiation and percutaneous coronary intervention -- 6. The 'golden rules' of percutaneous coronary intervention -- 7. Routine management after percutaneous coronary intervention -- <strong>Percutaneous coronary intervention-related imaging </strong> -- 8. Angiography: indications and limitations -- 9. Coronary physiology in clinical practice -- 10. The role of intravascular ultrasound in percutaneous coronary intervention -- 11. Virtual histology intravascular ultrasound and optical coherence tomography in percutaneous coronary intervention -- 12. Coronary computed tomography for the interventionalist -- 13. Cardiovascular magnetic resonance -- <strong>Percutaneous coronary intervention by clinical syndrome </strong> -- 14. Stable coronary artery disease: medical therapy versus percutaneous coronary intervention versus surgery -- 15. Percutaneous coronary intervention in non-ST elevation acute coronary syndrome -- 16. Primary percutaneous coronary intervention for ST elevation myocardial infarction -- 17. Percutaneous coronary intervention in patients with impaired left ventricular function -- <strong>Percutaneous coronary intervention by lesion and patient subsets </strong> -- 18. Coronary bifurcation stenting: state of the art -- 19. Percutaneous coronary intervention for unprotected and protected left main stem disease -- 20. Chronic total occlusions -- 21. Revascularization in diabetes mellitus -- <strong>Adjunctive therapies in percutaneous coronary intervention </strong> -- 22. Current status of oral antiplatelet therapies -- 23. Current status of glycoprotein IIb/IIIa inhibitors -- 24. The contemporary use of antiplatelet therapy in interventional cardiology -- 25. The role of bivalirudin in percutaneous coronary intervention -- 26. Optimal medical therapy in percutaneous coronary intervention patients: statins and ACE inhibitors as disease-modifying agents -- <strong>Complications of percutaneous coronary intervention </strong> -- 27. Contrast-induced acute kidney injury -- 28. In-stent restenosis in the drug-eluting stent era -- 29. Stent thrombosis -- 30. Stent loss and retrieval -- 31. No-reflow -- 32. Coronary artery perforation --

<strong>Special devices in percutaneous coronary intervention </strong> -- 33. Rotational atherectomy -- 34. Laser -- 35. Cutting balloons and AngioSculpt -- 36. Thrombus extraction in the contemporary management of ST-segment elevation myocardial infarction -- 37. Distal protection -- <strong>Non-coronary percutaneous interventions </strong> -- 38. Percutaneous device closure of atrial septal defect and patent foramen ovale -- 39. Transcatheter aortic valve replacement -- 40. Mitral balloon valvuloplasty -- 41. Alcohol septal ablation for obstructive hypertrophic cardiomyopathy -- 42. Carotid artery stenting.

| | |
|---|---|
| *Subjects* | Angioplasty. |
| | Coronary heart disease--Surgery. |
| | Cardiac catheterization. |
| | Cardiovascular Surgical Procedures. |
| | Cardiovascular Diseases--surgery. |
| *Notes* | Includes bibliographical references and index. |
| *Series* | Oxford textbooks in cardiology |
| | Oxford textbooks in cardiology. |

**Perioperative kidney injury: principles of risk assessment, diagnosis and treatment**

| | |
|---|---|
| *LCCN* | 2014944534 |
| *Type of material* | Book |
| *Main title* | Perioperative kidney injury: principles of risk assessment, diagnosis and treatment / Charuhas V. Thakar, Chirag R. Parikh, editors. |
| *Published/Produced* | New York: Springer, [2015] |
| *Description* | xvii, 251 pages: illustrations (some color); 24 cm |
| *ISBN* | 9781493912728 (alk. paper) |
| | 1493912720 (alk. paper) |
| *LC classification* | RC918.R4 P39 2015 |
| *Related names* | Thakar, Charuhas V., editor. |
| | Parikh, Chirag R., editor. |
| *Summary* | The kidneys participate in all vital processes of the body to maintain overall homeostasis and health. When kidneys are injured during surgical interventions, metabolic and hemodynamic control is |

disrupted, leading to dysfunction associated with greater mortality, length of hospital stay, and cost. Peri-operative Kidney Injury presents the epidemiology, risk factors, diagnosis, treatment, and outcomes associated with kidney injury during the peri-operative period. Concepts and principles of care to prevent kidney complications during surgical procedures are provided to equip health care professionals along with strategies to manage acute kidney injury and associated challenges when they occur. Chapters detail diverse surgical settings, ranging from the more common, such as abdominal, cardiac, and vascular surgeries, to the intricately complex, including the use of the left ventricular assist device and organ transplants. This practical and comprehensive text blends the evidence-based standards of care with cutting edge advances in the field, while also providing the reader with a peek into innovations on the horizon.

*Contents*

Part I Peri-operative AKI: Overview and Approach -- 1 Incidence, Trends and Diagnosis of Peri-operative AKI -- 2 Serious peri-operative complications: Hospital Medicine Perspectives -- 3 Role of Novel Kidney Injury Biomarkers in Perioperative AKI -- 4 Clinical Pearls: Renal Replacement Therapy for AKI in the Post-operative Period.- 5 Clinical Pearls: Non-dialytic Management of Kidney Complications in the Post-operative Period -- 6 Intra-Operative Considerations to Prevent Post-Operative AKI -- Part II Cardiac and Vascular Surgery -- 7 AKI after Cardiac Surgery in Adults.- 8 AKI after Cardiovascular Surgery in Children -- 9 AKI in the Era of Ventricular Assist Devices.- 10 Kidney Injury after Vascular Surgery.- Part III Abdominal and Urologic Surgery.- 11 AKI after Major Abdominal Surgery.- 12 Kidney Injury in Abdominal Compartment Syndrome.- 13 Kidney Function and Injury after Nephrectomy for Kidney Cancer -- Part IV Transplant Surgery -- 14 The Kidney in Non-Renal Solid Organ Transplantation -- 15 Acute

| | |
|---|---|
| | Allograft Injury After Kidney Transplantation -- Part V Special Topics in Peri-operative AKI.- 16 Trauma and Acute Kidney Injury -- 17 Fluid-Electrolyte Imbalances and Extra-Corporeal Therapy in the Neurosurgical Setting -- 18 Nutrition in Peri-operative Patients with Kidney Failure. |
| *Subjects* | Acute renal failure.<br>Medicine.<br>Anesthesiology.<br>Critical care medicine.<br>Nephrology.<br>Surgery.<br>Acute Kidney Injury--diagnosis.<br>Acute Kidney Injury--therapy.<br>Postoperative Complications.<br>Risk Factors.<br>Anesthesiology.<br>Critical care medicine.<br>Medicine.<br>Nephrology.<br>Surgery. |
| *Notes* | Includes bibliographical references and index. |

**Pharmacotherapy principles and practice**

| | |
|---|---|
| *LCCN* | 2010004385 |
| *Type of material* | Book |
| *Main title* | Pharmacotherapy principles and practice / editors, Marie A. Chisholm-Burns ... [et al.]. |
| *Edition* | 2nd ed. |
| *Published/Created* | New York: McGraw-Hill, c2010. |
| *Description* | xxxiv, 1869 p.: col. ill.; 29 cm. |
| *ISBN* | 9780071621809 (hardback: alk. paper)<br>0071621806 (hardback: alk. paper) |
| *LC classification* | RM262 .P475 2010 |
| *Other title* | Pharmacotherapy principles and practice |
| *Related names* | Chisholm-Burns, Marie A. |
| *Contents* | Introduction / Jack E. Fincham -- Geriatrics / Jeannie K. Lee ... [et al.] -- Pediatrics / Hanna Phan, Vinita B. Pai, Milap C. Nahata -- Palliative care / Marc A. |

Sweeney and Phyllis A. Grauer -- Hypertension / Robert J. Straka, David Parra, and Kade T. Birkeland -- Heart failure / Orly Vardeny and Tien M.H. Ng -- Ischemic heart disease / Larisa H. Cavallari and Robert J. DiDomenico -- Acute coronary syndromes / Sarah A. Spinler and Simon de Denus -- Arrhythmias / James E. Tisdale -- Venous thromboembolism / Edith A. Nutescu and Stuart T. Haines -- Stroke / Susan R. Winkler -- Dyslipidemias / Matthew K. Ito -- Hypovolemic shock / Bradley A. Boucher and G. Christopher Wood -- Asthma / W. Greg Leader -- Chronic obstructive pulmonary disease / Tara R. Whetsel and Nicole D. Verkleeren -- Cystic fibrosis / Kimberly J. Novak -- Gastroesophageal reflux disease / Dianne B. Williams and Marie A. Chishom-Burns -- Peptic ulcer disease / John W. Devlin -- Inflammatory bowel disease / Brian A. Hemstreet -- Nausea and vomiting / Sheila Wilhelm -- Constipation, diarrhea, and irritable bowel syndrome / Beverly C. Mims and Clarence E. Curry Jr. -- Portal hypertensio and cirrhosis / Laurajo Ryan -- Pancreatitis / Joseph J. Kishel -- Viral hepatitis / Juliana Chan -- Acute kidney injury / Mary K. Stamatakis -- Chronic and end-stage kidney diseases / Kristine S. Schonder -- Fluids and electrolytes / Mark A. Malesker and Lee E. Morrow -- Acid-base disturbances / Lee E. Morrow and Mark A. Malesker -- Epilepsy / Timothy E. Welty and Edward Faught -- Status epilepticus / Gretchen M. Brophy and Eljim P. Tesoro -- Parkinson's disease / Mary L. Wagner -- Pain management / Christine K. O'Neil -- Headache / Leigh Ann Ross and Brendan S. Ross -- Alzheimer's disease / Megan J. Ehret, Gary M. Levin, and Toya M. Bowles -- Substance-related disorders / Sally K. Guthrie and Theadia L. Carey -- Schizophrenia / Deanna L. Kelly, Elaine Weiner, and Heidi J. Wehring -- Major depressive disorder / Cherry W. Jackson, Marshall E. Cates, and Jacqueline M. Feldman -- Bipolar disorder / Brian L. Crabtree and Martha J. Faulkner -- Generalized anxiety disorder, panic idsorder, and social anxiety disorder / Sheila Botts, Anna Lockwood, and Timothy Allen -- Sleep disorders / John M. Dopp and Bradley G. Phillips -- Attention-deficit hyperactivity disorder / John Erramouspe and Kevin W. Cleveland -- Diabetes mellitus / John T. Johnson, Susan Cornell, and William E. Wade -- Thyroid disorders / Michael D. Katz -- Adrenal gland disorders / Devra K. Dang ... [et al.] -- Pituitary gland disorders / Judy T. Chen ... [et al.] -- Pregnancy and lactation: therapeutic considerations / Ema Ferreira, Évelyne Rey, and Caroline Morin -- Contraception / Julia M. Koehler and Kathleen B. Haynes -- Menstruation-related disorders / Elena M. Umland, Lara C. Weinstein, and Edward Buchanan -- Hormone therapy in menopause / Nicole S. Culhane and Kelly R. Ragucci -- Erectile dysfunction / Cara Liday and Catherine Heyneman -- Benign prostatic hyperplasia / Mary Lee and Roohollah Sharifi -- Urinary incontinence and pediatric enuresis / David R.P. Guay -- Allergic and pseudoallergic drug reactions / J. Russell May and Philip H. Smith -- Solid organ transplantation / Steven Gabardi and Ali J. Olyaei -- Osteoporosis / Beth Bryles Phillips -- Rheumatoid arthritis / Susan P. Bruce -- Osteoarthritis / Steven M. Smith, Benjamin J. Epstein, and John G. Gums -- Gout and hyperuricemia / Geoffrey C. Wall -- Musculoskeletal disorders / Jill S. Burkiewicz -- Glaucoma / Mikael D. Jones -- Allergic rhinitis / David A. Apgar -- Ophthalmic disorders / Kendra J. Grande -- Psoriasis / Rebecca M.T. Law -- Common skin disorders / Angie L. Goeser -- Anemia / Edward C. Li and James M. Hoffman -- Coagulation and platelet disorders / Anastasia Rivkin -- Sickle cell anemia / Tracy M. Hagemann and Teresa V. Lewis -- Antimicrobial regimen selection / Catherine M. Oliphant and Karl Madaras-Kelly -- Central nervous system infections / P. Brandon Bookstaver and April D. Miller -- Lower respiratory tract infections / Diane M. Cappelletty -- Upper respiratory tract infections /

| | |
|---|---|
| | Heather VandenBussche -- Skin and soft tissue infections / Christie Nelson, Jaime R. Hornecker, and Randy Wesnitzer -- Infective endocarditis / Ronda L. Akins -- Tuberculosis / Charles A. Peloquin and Rocsanna Namdar -- Gastrointestinal infections / Elizabeth D. Hermsen and Ziba Jalali -- Intra-abdominal infections / Joseph T. DiPiro and Thomas R. Howdieshell -- Parasitic diseases / J.V. Anandan -- Urinary tract infections / Kathryn R. Matthias and Brian A. Potoski -- Sexually transmitted infections / Marlon S. Honeywell and Michael D. Thompson -- Osteomyelitis / Melinda M. Neuhauser and Susan L. Pendland -- Sepsis and septic shock / S. Scott Sutton -- Superficial fungal infections / Lauren S. Schlesselman -- Invasive fungal infections / Russell E. Lewis and P. David Rogers -- Antimicrobial prophylaxis in surgery / Mary A. Ullman, Jeremy A. Schafer, and John C. Rotschafer -- Vaccines and toxoids / Marianne Billeter -- Human immunodeficiency virus infection / Amanda Corbett .. [et al.] --<br>Cancer chemotherapy and treatment / Dianne Brundage -- Breast cancer / Gerald Higa -- Lung cancer / Val Adams and Justin Balko -- Colorectal cancer / Patrick J. Medina -- Prostate cancer / Trevor McKibbin and Jill M. Kolesar -- Malignant lymphomas / Christopher Fausel and Patrick J. Kiel -- Ovarian cancer / Judith A. Smith -- Acute leukemia / Nancy Heideman -- Chronic leukemias and multiple myeloma / Amy M. Pick -- Skin cancer / Trinh Pham and Jennifer Nam Choi -- Hematopoietic stem cell transplantation / Amber P. Lawson -- Supportive care in oncology / Sarah L. Scarpace -- Parenteral nutrition / Michael D. Kraft and Imad F. Btaiche -- Enteral nutrition / Sarah J. Miller -- Overweight and obesity / Maqual R. Graham and Cameron C. Lindsey. |
| *Subjects* | Chemotherapy--Textbooks.<br>Drug Therapy. |
| *Notes* | Includes bibliographical references and index. |

**Renal and metabolic disorders**

| | |
|---|---|
| *LCCN* | 2012017048 |
| *Type of material* | Book |
| *Main title* | Renal and metabolic disorders / edited by John A. Kellum and Jorge Cerdá. |
| *Published/Created* | Oxford: Oxford University Press, c2013. |
| *Description* | xv, 222 p.; 21 cm. |
| *ISBN* | 9780199751600 (pbk.: acid-free paper) |
| *LC classification* | RC902 .R3665 2013 |
| *Related names* | Kellum, John A. |
| | Cerdá, Jorge, 1949- |
| *Contents* | AKI I: the critically ill patient -- Acute kidney injury in special circumstances -- AKI and sepsis -- The critically ill patient with chronic kidney disease -- Principles of fluid management -- Functional hemodynamic monitoring -- Pharmacologic therapy in acute kidney injury -- Drug dosing in kidney disease -- Renal Replacement therapy (RRT) indications, timing, and patient selection -- Choosing a Renal Replacement therapy in acute kidney injury -- Combined kidney-lung failure -- Acute kidney injury in cirrhosis -- Renal disorders in pregnancy -- Renal disorders in pediatrics -- Acid-base disorders -- Electrolyte disorders -- Management of the renal transplant patient in the ICU -- Diabetes mellitus -- Thyroid conditions in critical care -- Adrenal disease in critical care -- Calcium, bone, and mineral disease in the critically ill patient -- Nutrition in the critically ill patient. |
| *Subjects* | Kidney Diseases--therapy. |
| | Critical Care. |
| | Endocrine System Diseases--therapy. |
| | Metabolic Diseases--therapy. |
| *Notes* | Includes bibliographical references and index. |
| *Series* | Pittsburgh critical care medicine series |
| | Pittsburgh critical care medicine. |

**Renal disease in cancer patients**

| | |
|---|---|
| *LCCN* | 2014397035 |
| *Type of material* | Book |
| *Main title* | Renal disease in cancer patients / edited by Kevin W. Finkel, UTHealth Science Center-Medical School, Houston, TX, USA and University of Texas MD Anderson Cancer Center, Houston, TX, USA, Scott C. Howard, St. Jude Children's Research Hospital, Memphis, TN, USA. |
| *Published/Produced* | Amsterdam; Boston: Elsevier/AP, [2014] |
| *Description* | xviii, 293 pages, 16 unnumbered pages of plates: illustrations (some color); 25 cm |
| *ISBN* | 9780124159488 (hbk)<br>0124159486 (hbk) |
| *LC classification* | RC903 .R485 2014 |
| *Related names* | Finkel, Kevin W., editor.<br>Howard, Scott C., editor. |
| *Contents* | Introduction / Scott C. Howard, Kevin W. Finkel -- Acute kidney injury in cancer patients / Joseph R. Angelo, Joshua A. Samuels -- Biomarkers in oncology and nephrology / Putao Cen, [et al.] -- Tumor lysis syndrome / Scott C. Howard, Ching-Hon Pui, Raul C. Ribeiro -- Multiple myeloma and kidney disease / Amit Lahoti -- Kidney disease in patients undergoing hematopoietic cell transplantation / Benjamin L. Laskin, Sangeeta R. Hingorani -- Radiation-associated kidney injury / Amber S. Podoll, Mark J. Amsbaugh -- Molecular-targeted therapy for renal cell carcinoma / Robert J. Amato, Mika Stepankiw, Nwabugwu S. Ochuwa -- Renal tumors in children / Kelly L. Vallance, Jeffrey S. Dome -- Renal effects of leukemia and lymphoma / Kevin W. Finkel -- Fluid and electrolyte abnormalities in patients with cancer / Ala Abudayyeh, Maen Abdelrahim, Abdulla Salahudeen -- Infections of the kidney in cancer patients / Brett Stephens -- Drug nephropathies / Ilya G. Glezerman -- Paraneoplastic glomerulopathy / Sheron Latcha, Surya V. Seshan -- Pharmacokinetics of anti-cancer chemotherapy in renal insufficiency and dialysis / |

William H. Fissell IV, Marc Earl -- Cancer in renal transplant patients / Aleksandra M. De Golovine, Horacio E. Adrogue.

*Subjects* Kidneys--Diseases.
Cancer--Complications.
Kidney Diseases--complications.
Neoplasms--complications.

*Notes* Includes bibliographical references and index.

*Additional formats* Electronic version: (OCoLC)857711848

**Renal nursing**

*LCCN* 2013019908

*Type of material* Book

*Main title* Renal nursing / edited by Nicola Thomas.

*Edition* Fourth edition.

*Published/Produced* Chichester, West Sussex, UK: John Wiley and Sons Inc., 2014.

*ISBN* 9781118410646 (pbk.)

*LC classification* RC918.R4

*Related names* Thomas, Nicola, editor.

*Contents* The history of dialysis and transplantation -- Applied anatomy and physiology and the renal disease process -- Patient and carer involvement in renal nursing care, education and research -- Psychological perspectives -- Acute kidney injury -- Chronic kidney disease -- Investigations in kidney disease -- Haemodialysis -- Peritoneal dialysis -- Renal transplantation -- Non dialytic options and the role of palliative care -- Renal care in infancy, childhood and early adulthood -- Renal nutrition -- Quality improvement in renal nursing.

*Subjects* Kidney Diseases--nursing.

*Notes* Includes bibliographical references and index.

*Additional formats* Online version: Renal nursing Fourth edition. Chichester, West Sussex, UK: John Wiley and Sons Inc., 2014 9781118410721 (DLC) 2013020673

**Surgical critical care for the MRCS OSCE**

*LCCN* 2015012526

*Type of material* Book

| | |
|---|---|
| *Personal name* | Kanani, Mazyar, author. |
| *Uniform title* | Surgical critical care vivas |
| *Main title* | Surgical critical care for the MRCS OSCE / Mazyar Kanani, Phd, FRCS, Consultant Cardiothoracic Surgeon, Cardiac Unit, Great Ormond Street Hospital, London, UK, Simon Lammy, PgDip (Oxon), ST2 Neurological Surgery (Neurosurgery), Institute of Neurological Sciences, Southern General Hospital, Glasgow, UK. |
| *Edition* | Second edition. |
| *Published/Produced* | Cambridge, United Kingdom: Cambridge University Press, 2015. |
| *Description* | 315 pages: illustrations; 19 cm |
| *ISBN* | 9781107657687 (paperback: alk.) |
| *LC classification* | RC86.9 .K36 2015 |
| *Related names* | Lammy, Simon, author. |
| *Summary* | "Surgical practice has changed enormously since the first edition of Surgical Critical Care Vivas, as shown by the introduction of the MRCS Part B OSCE. This landmark book has been fully updated to reflect the latest NICE and SIGN guidelines and common ALS principles in critical care patients, as well as current ATLS® and CCrISP® guidelines (e.g., CT scanning in trauma). The alphabetical format of the previous edition is replaced by an ABCDE chapter format, incorporating an escalating level of diagnostic and management complexity in conjunction with a concise mini-bibliography in each chapter, enabling the reader to rapidly access the required information. Covering both non-ICU-based patients and basic fundamentals of ICU care, the chapters introduce standard definitions, pathological processes and diagnostic features, before discussing common investigations and suggested management plans. A must-have revision guide for all surgical trainees, from final year medical students through to junior surgical registrars"-- Provided by publisher. |
| *Contents* | Machine generated contents note: Acknowledgments; List of abbreviations; Ward Care (Levels 0-2): Part I. |

Airway: Section 1. Assessment: 1. Airway assessment; Section 2. Basic Concepts: 2. Oxygen: basic physiology; 3. Carbon dioxide: basic physiology; 4. Oxygen: therapy; 5. Oxygen monitoring (pulse oximetry); Section 3. Procedures: 6. Airway adjuncts; Part II. Breathing: Section 4. Assessment: 7. Respiratory assessment; Section 5. Basic Concepts: 8. Atelectasis; 9. Bronchiectasis; 10. Pneumonia; 11. Pneumothorax; Section 6. Complex Concepts: 12. Acute respiratory distress syndrome (ARDS); 13. Flail chest; 14. Pulmonary thromboembolism (PE); 15. Respiratory failure; Section 7. Procedures: 16. Chest drains: the surgical way; Part III. Circulation: Section 8. Assessment: 17. Cardiac assessment; Section 9. Basic Concepts: 18. Blood pressure monitoring; 19. Blood products; 20. Blood transfusion; 21. ECG: basic concepts; 22. ECG: complex concepts; 23. Fluid therapy; 24. Jugular venous pulse (JVP); Section 10. Complex Concepts: 25. Aortic dissection; 26. Cardiogenic shock; 27. Coagulation defects; 28. Disseminated intravascular coagulation; 29. Fat embolism syndrome; 30. Haemorrhagic shock; Section 11. Procedures: 31. Arterial lines: intra-arterial blood pressure monitoring; 32. Central access: central lines; Part IV. Disability (Neurological Evaluation): Section 12. Assessment: 33. Neurological assessment; Section 13. Basic Concepts: 34. Analgesia; Section 14. Complex Concepts: 35. Cerebral physiology: basic principles; 36. Cerebral pathophysiology: basic principles; 37. Spinal injury; Section 15. Procedures: 38. Lumbar puncture; Part V. Exposure (Everything Else): Section 16. Renal: 39. Acid-base balance; 40. Metabolic acidosis; 41. Metabolic alkalosis; 42. Lactic acidosis; 43. Electrolyte balance: calcium (and phosphate); 44. Electrolyte balance: magnesium; 45. Electrolyte balance potassium; 46. Electrolyte balance: sodium; 47. Oliguria: low urine output state; 48. Renal failure: acute kidney injury (AKI); 49. Renal failure: chronic kidney disease (CKD); Section 17. Other

| | |
|---|---|
| | Systemic Processes: 50. Burns; 51. Nutrition: basic concepts; 52. Nutrition: enteral; 53. Nutrition: parenteral (TPN); 54. Rhabdomyolysis; 55. Systemic response to trauma; Intensive Care (Level 3): Part VI. Intensive Care Unit: Section 18. Assessment: 56. Agitation and sedation; Section 19. Complex Concepts: 57. Brainstem death and organ donation; 58. Circulatory support: inotropic agents; 59. Endotracheal intubation; 60. Extubation and weaning; 61. ICU admission criteria; 62. Mechanical ventilation and support; 63. Pulmonary artery catheters; 64. Renal replacement therapy; 65. Septic shock; 66. Transfer of the critically ill patient; Section 20. Procedures: 67. Tracheostomy; Index. |
| *Subjects* | Critical Care--Examination Questions.<br>Surgical Procedures, Operative--Examination Questions. |
| *Notes* | Preceded by: Surgical critical care vivas / Mazyar Kanani. 2003.<br>Includes bibliographical references and index. |

**Textbook of post-ICU medicine: the legacy of critical care**

| | |
|---|---|
| *LCCN* | 2014931564 |
| *Type of material* | Book |
| *Main title* | Textbook of post-ICU medicine: the legacy of critical care / edited by Robert D. Stevens, MD, Associate Professor of Anesthesiology Critical Care Medicine, Associate Professor of Neurology, Neurosurgery and Radiology, Johns Hopkins University School of Medicine, F.M. Kirby Center for Functional Brain imaging, Kennedy Krieger Institute, Baltimore, Maryland, Nicholas Hart, MBBS, BSc, MRCP, FFICM, Clincal and Academic Director, Lane Fox Respiratory Unit, St Thomas' Hospital, Guy's and St Thomas NHS Foudation Trust, London, UK, Reader in Respiratory and Critical Care Medicine, Department of Asthma, Allergy and Respiratory Science, Division of Asthma, Allergy and Lung Biology, King's College London, London, UK, Margaret S. Herridge, MSc, |

MD, FRCPC, MPH, Professor of Medicine, University of Toronto, Critical Care and Pulmonary Medicine Scientist, Toronto General Research Institute, University Health Network/Toronto General Hospital NCSB 11C-1180, Toronto, ON, Canada.

*Edition* First edition.

*Published/Produced* Oxford, United Kingdom; New York, NY, United States of America: Oxford University Press, 2014.

*Description* xxiv, 624 pages: illustrations (black and white); 26 cm.

*ISBN* 9780199653461 (hardback)
0199653461 (hardback)

*LC classification* RC86.7 .T456 2014

*Variant title* Textbook of post-Intensive Care Unit medicine

*Related names* Stevens, Robert D., editor.
Hart, Nicholas (Physician), editor.
Herridge, Margaret S., editor.

*Contents* Machine generated contents note: pt. 1 Life after the ICU -- 1. Introduction: Life after the ICU / Margaret S. Herridge -- 2. Critical Illness and Long-Term Outcomes Worldwide / Neill K.J. Adhikari -- 3. Mortality after Critical Illness / Hannah Wunsch -- 4. The Role of Long-Term Ventilator Hospitals / Jeremy M. Kahn -- 5. The Overlap of Palliative Care and Critical Illness / Judith E. Nelson -- 6. Patterns of Recovery after Critical Illness / Theodore J. Iwashyna -- 7. Quality of Life after Critical Illness / Peter E. Spronk -- 8. Costs and Resource Utilization in Prolonged Critical Illness / Christopher E. Cox -- 9. Caring for the ICU survivor: The Family Caregiver Burden / Mark D. Siegel -- 10. Survival and Recovery: A Patients Perspective / Cheryl Misak -- 11. One Family's Perspective on the Legacy of Critical Illness / David Dyzenhaus -- pt. 2 Chronic Organ Dysfunction Following Critical Illness -- 12. Introduction: Chronic Organ Dysfunction Following Critical Illness / Greet Hermans. 13. Chronic Multiple Organ Dysfunction / Shannon S. Carson -- 14. Prolonged Respiratory Insufficiency and Ventilator Dependence in the ICU / Laurent Brochard -- 15. The Long-Term Outcomes of

Acute Kidney Injury / Ziv Harel -- 16. Severe Burn Injuries and Their Long-Term Implications / David N. Herndon -- 17. Consequences of Endotracheal Intubation and Tracheostomy / Stefan Kluge -- pt. 3 Cognitive and Behavioural Disorders Following Critical Illness -- 18. Introduction: Cognitive and Behavioural Disorders Following Critical Illness / E. Wesley Ely -- 19. Cognitive Impairment Following Critical Illness / James C. Jackson -- 20. Depressive Mood States Following Critical Illness / O. Joseph Bienvenu -- 21. Post-Traumatic Stress Disorder Following Critical Illness / Richard D. Griffiths -- 22. Sleep Disorders and Recovery from Critical Illness / Nancy A. Collop -- pt. 4 Neuromuscular and Musculoskeletal Disorders Following Critical Illness. 23. Introduction: Neuromuscular and Musculoskeletal Disorders Following Critical Illness / Naeem A. Ali -- 24. Long-Term Implications of ICU-Acquired Muscle Weakness / Victoria McCredie -- 25. Bone and Joint Disease Following Critical Illness / Guy Trudel -- pt. 5 Biological Mechanisms of Injury and Repair -- 26. Introduction: Biological Mechanisms of Injury and Repair / Robert D. Stevens -- 27. Genetic Determinants of Sepsis Outcomes / Derek C. Angus -- 28. Physiological Reserve and Frailty in Critical Illness / Sean M. Bagshaw -- 29. Cognitive Reserve / Robert D. Stevens -- 30. Pathophysiology of Acute Kidney Injury, Repair, and Regeneration / Hamid Rabb -- 31. Myocardial Remodelling after Myocardial Infarction / Michael Marber -- 32. Sepsis-Associated Encephalopathy / Tarek Sharshar -- 33. Critical Illness Neuropathy, Myopathy, and Sodium Channelopathy / Mark M. Rich -- 34. The Impact of Critical Illness on Skeletal Muscle Structure / Catherine L. Hough. 35. Skeletal Muscle Mass Regulation in Critical Illness / Stephen Harridge -- 36. Malnutrition in Critical Illness: Implications, Causes, and Therapeutic Approaches / Marina Mourtzakis -- pt. 6 Therapeutic and Rehabilitation Strategies in the ICU -- 37.

Introduction: Therapeutic and Rehabilitation Strategies in the ICU / Nicholas Hart -- 38. Choice of Renal Replacement Therapy and Renal Recovery / Rinaldo Bellomo -- 39. Ventilator Liberation Strategies / Luca Fasano -- 40. Rethinking Sedation in the ICU / Sangeeta Mehta -- 41. Sleep-Promoting Strategies / V. Marco Ranieri -- 42. Effects of Insulin and Glycaemic Management on Neuromuscular Function / Greet Hermans -- 43. Physical and Occupational Therapy in the ICU / John P. Kress -- 44. Neuromuscular Electrical Stimulation: A New Therapeutic and Rehabilitation Strategy in the ICU / Serafim N. Nanas -- 45. Exercise and Early Rehabilitation in the Intensive Care Unit / Rik Gosselink. pt. 7 Therapeutic and Rehabilitation Strategies in the Post-ICU Period -- 46. Introduction: Therapeutic and Rehabilitation Strategies in the Post-ICU Period / Richard D. Griffiths -- 47. Assessment of Peripheral and Respiratory Muscle Strength in ICU / John Moxham -- 48. Clinical Pathways for the Continuum of Rehabilitation / Stephen Brett -- 49. Prolonged Weaning / Nicholas Hart -- 50. Models of Rehabilitative Care after Critical Illness / Jill I. Cameron -- 51. Post-ICU Rehabilitation / Linda Denehy -- 52. Narratives of Illness and Healing after the ICU / Christina Jones -- 53. ICU Follow-up Clinics / Brian H. Cuthbertson.

*Subjects*
Critical care medicine.
Intensive care nursing.
Intensive care units.
Intensive Care.
Critical Care.
Treatment Outcome.
Critical care medicine--Complications.
Intensivmedizin.
Intensivtherapie.
Nachsorge.
Rehabilitationsmedizin.

*Notes*
Formerly CIP.

Includes bibliographical references and index.

**The 5-minute pediatric consult**

| | |
|---|---|
| *LCCN* | 2012012664 |
| *Type of material* | Book |
| *Main title* | The 5-minute pediatric consult / editor, M. William Schwartz; associate editors, Louis M. Bell, Jr. ... [et al.]; assistant editor, Charles I. Schwartz. |
| *Edition* | 6th ed. |
| *Published/Created* | Philadelphia: Wolters Kluwer/Lippincott Williams and Wilkins, c2012. |
| *Description* | xxx, 1113 p.: ill.; 28 cm. |
| *ISBN* | 9781451116564 (hardback: alk. paper)<br>145111656X (hardback: alk. paper) |
| *LC classification* | RJ48 .A15 2012 |
| *Variant title* | Five-minute pediatric consult |
| *Related names* | Schwartz, M. William, 1935- |
| *Summary* | "The 5 Minute Pediatric Consult provides immediate, practical advice on problems seen in infants, children, and adolescents. More than 450 diseases and conditions are covered in the fast-access two-page outline format that makes The 5-Minute Consult Series titles so popular among busy clinicians. Other features include a Chief Complaints section addressing the workup and treatment of 50 signs and symptoms, plus a medication index, syndromes glossary, surgical glossary, laboratory values, and tables all for quick reference saving you time and helping to treat your patients more efficiently.In this sixth edition, the 5 Minute Pediatric Consult also offers free 30 day access to the 5minuteconsult Pediatric website -- a clinical decision support tool -- that can be accessed by the health care providers to address questions on-the-go via website or mobile.New Features: New topics for this edition include: Amenorrhea, Asberger Syndrome, Dental Trauma, Head banging, Mental Retardation, Narcolepsy, Obsessive Compulsive Disorder, Separation Anxiety and Social Anxiety Free 30 Day Access to the 5minuteconsult Pediatric Website |

Includes More than 450 diseases and conditions to support your patient care decisions Patient education handouts from AAP to help educate your patients Hundreds of Images from Chung's "Visual Diagnosis and Treatment in Pediatrics" and other reputable sources to provide you with quick visual guidance Immunization schedules and charts at your fingertips to save you time from searching Content is optimized for handheld devices so you have access to the content anytime, anywhere Updates to content made on a regular basis to keep you abreast of the latest content Visit 5minuteconsult.com and click on the "go to pediatric consult tab" to learn more about your free access and begin using today!"-- Provided by publisher.

*Contents* Abdominal Mass -- Abdominal migraine -- Abdominal pain -- Abnormal bleeding -- Acetaminophen poisoning -- Acne -- Acquired hypothyroidism -- Acute drug withdrawal -- Acute kidney injury -- Acute lymphoblastic leukemia -- Acute myeloid leukemia -- Adenovirus infection -- Alcohol (ethanol) intoxication -- Allergic child -- Alopecia (hair loss) -- Alpha-1-Antitrypsin defficiency -- Altitude illness -- Amblyopia -- Amebiasis -- Amenorrhea -- Anearobic infections -- Anaphylaxis -- Anemia of chronic disease (Anemia of inflammation) -- Anicryptococcal infections -- Ankylosing spondylitis -- Anomalous coronary artery -- Anorexia nervosa -- Anthrax -- Aplastic anemia -- Appendicitis -- Arthritis, Juvenile idiopathic (Rheumatoid) -- Ascaris lumbricoides -- Ascites -- Aspergillosis -- Asplenia/Hyposplenia -- Asthma -- Ataxia -- Atelectasis -- Atopic dermatitis -- Atrial septal defect -- Attention-Deficit/Hyperactivity disorder (ADHD) -- Atypical Mycobacterial infections -- Autism/Pervasive developmental disorder (PDD) Spectrum -- Autoimmune hemolytic anemia -- Avascular (aseptic) necrosis of the femoral head (HIP) -- Babesiosis -- Back pain -- Barotitis -- Bell palsy -- Bezoars -- Biliary Atresia -- Blastomycosis --

Blepharitis -- Bone marrow and stem cell transplant -- Botulism -- Brain abscess -- Brain injury, Traumatic -- Brain tumor -- Branchial cleft malformations -- Breast Abscess -- Breastfeeding -- Breastfeeding Jaundice and breast milk jaundice -- Breath-holding spells -- Bronchiolitis (See also: Respiratory syncytial virus) -- Bronchopulmonary dysplasia (Chronic lung disease of prematurity) -- Bruising -- Bruxism -- Bulimia -- C 1 Esterase inhibitor deficiency -- Campylobacter infections -- Candidiasis -- Carbon monoxide poisoning -- Cardimyopathy -- Cataract -- Cat-scratch disease -- Cavernous Sinus Syndrome -- Cavernous transformation and portal vein obstruction -- Celiac disease -- Cellulitis -- Cerebral palsy -- Cervicitis -- Chancroid -- Chest Pain -- Chickenpox) Varicella, Herpes Zoster) -- Child abuse, Physical -- Chlamydial infections -- Cholelithiasis -- Cholera -- Chronic Diarrhea -- Chronic granulmatous disease -- Chronic hepatitis -- Chronic kidney disease -- Cirrhosis -- Cleft lip and palate -- Clubfoot -- Coarctation of aorta -- Coccidioidomycosis -- Colic -- Coma -- Common variable immunodeficiency -- Complement deficiency -- Concussion -- Congenital hepatic fibrosis -- Congenital hypothyroidism -- Congestive heart failure -- Conjunctivitis -- Constipation -- Contact Dermatitis -- Contraception -- Cor pulmonale -- Costochondritis -- Cough -- Crohn disease -- Croup -- Crying -- Cryptococcal infections -- Cryptorchidism -- Cryptosporidiosis -- Cushing Syndrome (Adrenal Excess) -- Cutaneous Larva Migrans -- Cyclospora -- Cystic fibrosis -- Cytomegalovirus infection --22q11.2 Deletion Syndrome (Digeorge Syndrome) -- Dental/Oral Pain and urgencies -- Dermatomyositis/ Polymyositis -- Developmental disabilities -- Developmental dysplasia of the hip -- Diabetes insipidus -- Diabetes mellitus -- Diabetic ketoacidosis -- Diaper rash -- Diaphragmatic hernia (Congenital) -- Diarrhea -- Diphtheria -- Diskitis -- Disorders of sex development -- Disseminated intravascular coagulation

-- Down (Trisomy 21) Syndrome -- Drowning -- Dysfunctional uterine bleeding -- Dysmenorrhea -- Dyspnea -- Dysuria -- Earache -- Edema -- Ehrlichiosis and anaplasmosis -- Encephalitis -- Encopresis -- Endocarditis -- Enuresis -- Endocarditis -- Epiglottitis -- Epstein Barr virus (Infectious Mononucleosis -- Erythema multiforme -- Erythema Nodosum -- Ewing Sarcoma -- Exstrophy of the bladder, cloacal exstrophy, and epispadias -- Failure to thrive -- Feeding disorders -- Fetal alcohol syndrome -- Fever and petechiae -- Fever of unknown cause -- Floppy infant syndrome -- Food allergy -- Food poisoning or foodborne illness -- Fragile X syndrome -- Frostbite -- Functional diarrhea of infancy or toddLer's diarrhea -- Fungal skin infections (Dermatophyte infections, Candidiasis, and Tinea Versicolor) -- Gastritis -- Gastroesophageal reflux -- German measles (third disease, Rubella) -- Giardiasis -- Gingivitis -- Glaucoma--congenital -- Glomerulonephritis -- Gluecose-6-phosphate dehydrogenase deficiency -- Goiter -- Gonococcal infections -- Graft versus host disease -- Graves disease -- Growth hormone deficiency -- Guillain-Barre syndrome -- Gynecomastia -- Hand, foot, and mouth disease -- Hantavirus -- Head banging -- Headache and migraine -- Heat stroke and related illness -- Hemangiomas and other vascular lesions -- Hematuria -- Hemolysis -- Hemolysis -- Hemolytic disease of the newborn -- Hemolytic uremic syndrome -- Hemophilia -- Hemoptysis -- Henoch-Schonlein purpura -- Hepatic failure -- Hepatomegaly -- Hereditary Angioedema -- Hereditary spherocytosis -- Heroin intoxication -- Herpes simplex virus -- Hiccups -- Hirschsprung disease -- Histiocytosis -- Histoplasmosis -- Hodgkin Lymphoma -- Human immunodeficiency virus infection -- Human papilloma virus -- Hydrocephalus -- Hydronephrosis -- Hyperimmunoglobulinemia E Syndrome -- Hyperinsulinism -- Hyperlipidemia -- Hypertention -- Hypogrammaglobulinemia --

Hypoparathyroidism -- Hypoplastic left heart syndrome -- Hypospadias -- Idiopathic intracranial hypertension (Pseudotumor cerebri) -- Idiopathic Thrombocytopenic purpura -- Immune deficiency -- Immunoglobulin a deficiency -- Imperforate anus -- Impetigo -- In Inappropriate antidiuretic hormone secretion -- Infantile spasms -- Influenza -- Inguinal hernia -- Intestinal obstruction -- Intoeing-tibial torsion -- Intracranial hemorrhage -- Intussusception -- Iron deficiency anemia -- Iron poisoning -- Irritable bowel syndrome -- Jaundice -- Kawasaki disease -- Knee pain, Anterior/Patellofemoral malalignment syndrome -- Lacrimal duct obstruction -- Lactos intolerance -- Lead poisoning -- Learning disabilities -- Luekocytosis -- Lice (Pediculosis) -- Lower GI bleeding -- Lupus erythematosus -- Lyme disease -- Lymphadenopathy -- Malabsorption -- Malaria -- Mammalian bites -- Mastoiditis -- Measles (Rubeola, first disease) -- Meckel diverticulum -- Mediastinal mass -- Megaloblastic anemia -- Meningitis -- Meningococcemia -- Mental retardation -- Mesenteric adenitis -- Metabolic diseases in hypoglycemic newborns -- Metabolic diseases in acidotic newborns -- Metabolic diseases in Hyperammonemic newborns -- Metabolic syndrome -- Methemoglobinemia -- Microcytic anemia -- Milia -- Milk protein intolerance -- Mumps/Parotitis -- Munchausen syndrome by proxy -- Muscular dystrophies -- Myasthenia gravis -- Myocarditis -- Narcolepsy -- Neck masses -- Necrotizing entercolitis -- Neonatal alloimmune thrombocytopenia -- Neonatal apnea -- Neonatal cholestasis -- Nephrotic syndrome -- Neural tube defects -- Neuroblastoma -- Neurofibromatosis -- Neutropenia -- Non-Hodgkin Lymphoma -- Nosebleeds (Epistaxis) -- Obesity -- Obsessive compulsive disorder -- Obstetric brachial plexus (ERB) palsy -- Omphalitis -- Osteogenesis imperfecta -- Osteosarcoma -- Osteomyelitis -- Otitis externa -- Otitis media -- Pallor -- Pancreatic Pseudocyst --

Pancreatitis -- Panhypopituitarism -- Parvovirus B 19 (Erythema Infectiosum, fifth disease) -- Patent ductus arteriosus -- Pelvic inflammatory disease (PID) -- Penile and foreskin problems -- Pericarditis -- Periodic breathing -- Periorbital cellulitis -- Perirectal abscess -- Peritonitis -- Peritonsillar abscess -- Persistent Pulmonary Hypertension of the newborn (PPHN) -- Perthes disease -- Pertussis -- Pharyngitis -- Photosensitivity -- Pinworms -- Plague -- Pleural effusion -- Pneumoystic Jiroveci (Previously known as Pneumocystic Carnii Pneumonis) -- Pneumonia-- Bacterial -- Pneumothorax -- Polyarteritis Nodosa -- Polycystic kidney disease -- Polycystic ovary syndrome -- Polycythemia -- Polyps, intestinal -- Porencephaly cortical dysplasia/neuronal migration disorders-malformations of cortical development -- Portal hypertension -- Posterior urethral valve -- Premature adrenarche -- Premature thelarche -- Premenstrual syndrome (PMS) -- Primary adrenal insufficiency -- Prion diseases (Transmissible spongiform encephalophathies) -- Probiotics -- Prolonged QT interval syndrome -- Protein-Energy malnutrition (Kwashiorkor) -- Proteinuria -- Prune belly syndrome -- Pruritus -- Psittacosis -- Psoriasis -- Pubertal delay -- Pulmonary embolism -- Pulmonary hypertension -- Purpura fulminans -- Pyelonephritis -- Pyloric stenosis -- Rabies -- Rectal prolapse -- Refractive error -- Renal artery stenosis -- Renal tubular acidosis -- Renal venous thrombosis -- Respiratory syncytial virus (RSV) -- Retinoblastoma -- Retropharyngeal abscess -- Reye Syndrome -- Rhabdomyolysis -- Rhabdomyosarcoma -- Rheumatic fever -- Rhinitis, Allergic -- Rickets -- Rickettsial disease -- Rocky Mountain Spotted Fever -- Roseola -- Rotavirus -- Salicylate poisoning (Aspirin) -- Salmonella infections -- Sarcoidosis -- Scabies -- Scarlet fever -- Scleroderma -- Scoliosis (Idiopathic) -- Seborrheic dermatitis -- Seizures-febrile -- Seizures, partial and generalized -- Separation anxiety disorder -

- Sepsis -- Septic arthritis -- Serum Sickness -- Severe acute respiratory syndrome (SARS) -- Severe combined immunodeficiency -- Sexual abuse -- Sexual ambiguity -- Sexual precocity -- Short-bowel syndrome -- Short stature -- Sickle cell disease -- Sinusitis -- Sleep apnea--obstructive sleep apnea syndrome -- Slipped capital femoral epiphysis -- Smallpox (Variola virus) -- Snake and insect bites -- Social anxiety disorder -- Sore throat -- Speech delay -- Speech problems -- Spinal muscular atrophy -- Splenomegaly -- Staphylococcal scaled skin syndrome (SSSS) -- Status epilepticus -- Stevens-Johnson syndrome and toxic epidermal necrolysis -- Stomatitis -- Strabismus -- Strep infection: invasive Group A Ç-hemolytic streptococcus -- Stroke -- Stuttering -- Subdural hematoma -- Substance use disorders -- Sudden Infant Death Syndrome (SIDS) -- Suicide -- Superior Mesenteric Artery syndrome -- Superior Mesenteric artery syndrome -- Supraventricular tachycardia -- Sympathomimetic poisoning -- Syncope -- Synovitis--transient -- Syphilis -- Tapeworm -- Teething -- Tendonitis -- Teratoma -- Tenanus -- Tetralogy of Fallot -- Thalassemia -- Thoracic insufficiency syndrome -- Thrombosis -- Tick fever -- Tics -- Toxic alcohols -- Toxic Shock syndrome -- Toxoplasmosis -- Tracheitis -- Tracheoesophageal fistula and esophageal atresia -- Tracheomalacia/laryngomalacia -- Transfusion reaction -- Transient erythroblastopenia of childhood -- Transient Trachypnea of the Newborn (TTN) -- Transposition of the great arteries -- Transverse myelitis -- Trichinosis -- Tuberculosis -- Tuberous sclerosis complex -- Tularemia -- Ulcerative colitis -- Upper gastrointestional bleeding -- Ureteropelvic junction obstruction -- Urethral prolapse -- Urinary tract infection -- Urticaria -- Vaccine adverse events -- Vaginitis -- Vascular brain lesions (Congenial) -- Ventricular septal defect -- Ventricular tachycardia -- Vesicoureteral reflux -- Viral hepatitis -- Volvulus --

| | |
|---|---|
| | Vomiting -- Von Willebrand disease -- Warts -- Weight loss -- West Nile Virus (And other Arbovirus Encephalitis) -- Wheezing -- Wilms tumor -- Wilson disease -- Wiskott-Aldrich syndrome -- Yersinia enterocolitica. |
| *Subjects* | Pediatrics--Handbooks, manuals, etc.<br>Pediatrics.<br>Pediatrics--Handbooks. |
| *Notes* | Includes bibliographical references and index. |
| *Series* | 5-minute consult series<br>5-minute consult. |

**The renal system: basic science and clinical conditions**

| | |
|---|---|
| *LCCN* | 2009017306 |
| *Type of material* | Book |
| *Personal name* | Field, Michael J. (Michael John), 1950- |
| *Main title* | The renal system: basic science and clinical conditions / Michael J. Field, Carol A. Pollock, David C. Harris; illustrations by Robert Britton. |
| *Edition* | 2nd ed. |
| *Published/Created* | Edinburgh; New York: Churchill Livingstone/Elsevier, 2010. |
| *Description* | 169 p.: ill.; 28 cm. |
| *ISBN* | 9780702033711 (alk. paper)<br>0702033715 (alk. paper) |
| *LC classification* | RC900 .F53 2010 |
| *Related names* | Pollock, Carol A.<br>Harris, David C. (David Charles), 1953- |
| *Contents* | Urinary tract structure and infection -- Body fluids, nephron function and diuretics -- Water balance and regulation of osmolality -- Acid-base balance and regulation of pH -- Glomerular filtration and acute kidney injury -- Proteinuria and the nephrotic syndrome -- Glomerulonephritis and the acute nephritic syndrome -- Diabetic nephropathy and chronic kidney disease -- End-stage kidney disease and replacement of renal function -- Hypertension and the kidney -- Pregnancy and the kidney -- Urinary tract obstruction and stones -- Renal masses and urinary |

| | |
|---|---|
| | tract tumours -- Drugs and the kidney. |
| *Subjects* | Urinary organs--Diseases.<br>Kidneys--Diseases.<br>Urologic Diseases--diagnosis--Problems and Exercises.<br>Diagnosis, Differential--Problems and Exercises.<br>Diagnostic Techniques, Urological--Problems and Exercises.<br>Urinary Tract Physiological Phenomena--Problems and Exercises. |
| *Notes* | Includes index. |
| *Series* | Systems of the body<br>Systems of the body. |

**Ultrasound imaging in acute and chronic kidney disease**

| | |
|---|---|
| *LCCN* | 2016015847 |
| *Type of material* | Book |
| *Main title* | Ultrasound imaging in acute and chronic kidney disease / volume editors Mario Meola, Ilaria Petrucci, Claudio Ronco. |
| *Published/Produced* | Basel; New York: Karger, 2016. |
| *ISBN* | 9783318058833 (hard cover: alk. paper) |
| *LC classification* | RC918.R4 |
| *Related names* | Meola, Mario, editor.<br>Petrucci, Ilaria, editor.<br>Ronco, C. (Claudio), 1951- editor. |
| *Contents* | Pathophysiology and clinical work-up of acute kidney injury / Meola, M., Nalesso, F., Petrucci, I., Samoni, S., Ronco, C -- Ultrasound in acute kidney disease / Meola, M., Nalesso, F., Petrucci, I., Samoni, S., Ronco, C -- Clinical scenarios in acute kidney injury: pre-renal acute kidney injury / Meola, M., Nalesso, F., Petrucci, I., Samoni, S., Ronco, C -- Clinical scenarios in acute kidney injury: hepato-renal syndrome / Meola, M., Nalesso, F., Petrucci, I., Samoni, S., Ronco, C -- Clinical scenarios in acute kidney injury: parenchymal acute kidney injury tubulo-interstitial diseases / Meola, M., Samoni, S., Petrucci, I., Ronco, C -- Clinical scenarios in acute kidney injury-parenchymal acute |

| | |
|---|---|
| | kidney injury, vascular diseases / Meola, M., Samoni, S., Petrucci, I., Ronco, C -- Clinical scenarios in acute kidney injury: post-renal acute kidney injury / Meola, M., Samoni, S., Petrucci, I., Ronco, C -- Imaging in chronic kidney disease / Meola, M., Samoni, S., Petrucci, I -- Clinical scenarios in chronic kidney disease: vascular chronic diseases / Meola, M., Samoni, S., Petrucci, I -- Clinical scenarios in chronic kidney disease: parenchymal chronic renal diseases, part 1 / Petrucci, I., Samoni, S., Meola, M -- Clinial scenarios in chronic kidney disease: parenchymal chronic renal diseases, part 2 / Petrucci, I., Samoni, S., Meola, M -- Clinical scenarios in chronic kidney disease: chronic tubulointerstitial diseases / Meola, M., Samoni, S., Petrucci, I -- Clinical scenarios in chronic kidney disease: cystic renal diseases / Meola, M., Samoni, S., Petrucci, I -- Clinical scenarios in chronic kidney disease: kidneys' structural changes in end stage renal disease / Meola, M., Samoni, S., Petrucci, I. |
| *Subjects* | Renal Insufficiency, Chronic--ultrasonography<br>Acute Kidney Injury--ultrasonography |
| *Notes* | Includes bibliographical references and index. |
| *Series* | Contributions to nephrology; vol. 188<br>Contributions to nephrology; v. 188. |

**Understanding the essentials of critical care nursing**

| | |
|---|---|
| *LCCN* | 2012005634 |
| *Type of material* | Book |
| *Personal name* | Perrin, Kathleen Ouimet. |
| *Main title* | Understanding the essentials of critical care nursing / Kathleen Ouimet Perrin, Carrie Edgerly MacLeod. |
| *Edition* | 2nd ed. |
| *Published/Created* | Boston: Pearson, c2013. |
| *Description* | xx, 579 p.: ill. (some col.); 28 cm. |
| *ISBN* | 9780132724159 (pbk.)<br>0132724154 (pbk.) |
| *LC classification* | RT120.I5 P47 2013 |
| *Related names* | MacLeod, Carrie Edgerly. |
| *Contents* | What is critical care? -- Care of critical ill patients -- |

| | |
|---|---|
| | Respiratory failure -- Interpretation and management of basic dysrhythmias -- Cardiodynamics/ hemodynamics -- Shock -- Heart failure -- Acute coronary syndrome -- Traumatic injury -- Intracranial dysfunction -- Cerebral or cerbrovascular disorder -- Alcohol withdrawal and liver failure -- Acute gastrointestinal bleed of pancreatitis -- Care of the patient with problems in glucose metabolism -- Care of the patient with acute kidney injury -- Transplant -- Burn patient -- Sepsis -- End of life. |
| *Subjects* | Critical Care--methods.<br>Critical Illness--nursing.<br>Nursing Care--methods. |
| *Notes* | Includes bibliographical references and index. |

# RELATED NOVA PUBLICATIONS

## ACUTE KIDNEY INJURY DUE TO INTRATUBULAR DEPOSITS OF ENDOGENOUS PIGMENTS: MYOGLOBINURIA AND HEMOGLOBINURIA*

***Consolación Rosado Rubio[1,†], Alberto Domínguez Bravo[2] and María López Veloso[3]***

[1]Complejo Asistencial de Ávila, España
[2]Servicio de Salud del Principado de Asturias, España
[3]Centre Hospitalier Tarbes-Lourdes, France

The deposit of endogenous pigments withing the kidney tubules can lead to renal failure, which will be acute or chronic depending on whether the renal damage is sustained over time. The typical example of these diseases is myoglobinuria, produced as a result of rhabdomyolysis and hemoglobinuria, secondary to intravascular hemolysis. Rhabdomyolysis is the injury that causes the breakdown of the cell membrane of the striated muscle, resulting in the release of the intracelular material into the extracellular fluid. Its causes are

* The full version of this chapter can be found in *Renal Failure: Diagnosis, Management and Potential Complications*, edited by Masayoshi Yamaguchi, published by Nova Science Publishers, Inc, New York, 2016.

† Correspondence author: Consolación Rosado Rubio, Complejo Asistencial de Ávila, España. E-mail: crosadorubio@hotmail.com

varied, being the most important: excessive physical activity, alcohol or drugs such as statins, prolonged immobilization or muscle crush syndrome. The main substance released is myoglobin, which has a nephrotoxic potential, but not enough to cause acute kidney damage, so the coexistence of volume depletion or renal hypoperfusion is necessary. The coexistence of these two factors produces several injuries in the kidney: renal vasoconstriction, intratubular obstruction by pigmentary casts and myoglobin direct cytotoxicity on renal structures. Thus, when the acute renal failure secondary to rhabdomyolysis occurs, morbidity and mortality increases significantly. Management comprises avoid or eliminate the triggering cause at an early stage and early aggressive hydration (it has been shown to be one of the most effective measures). Other measures to counteract the toxic effects of renal myoglobin have also been tested, with different success, as the use of bicarbonate or mannitol. Intravascular hemolysis can also induce acute renal failure through the release of heme pigments. This type of acute renal failure occurs in over 50% of cases of massive hemolysis, which may be due to different causes, both intrinsic and extrinsic to the red cells: hemoglobinopathies, membrane defects, prosthesic heart valves, hemolytic anemia and hypersplenism. The pathophysiology of renal damage, its prevention and treatment are similar to the kidney damage caused by myoglobin.

## Contrast-Induced Acute Kidney Injury*

***Vincenzo Barbera*† *and Antonio Gorini***

Department of Nephrology and Dialysis,
Colleferro County Hospital, Colleferro, Rome, Italy

Contrast-Induced Acute Kidney Injury (CI-AKI) represents a relevant cause of mortality and morbidity in patients after diagnostic and interventional

---

* The full version of this chapter can be found in *Comorbidities in Chronic Kidney Disease: From Diagnosis to Management*, edited by Luca Di Lullo, published by Nova Science Publishers, Inc, New York, 2016.

† Correspondence to: V. Barbera, Department of Nephrology and Dialysis. Colleferro County Hospital, Piazza Aldo Moro, 1 Colleferro, Rome, Italy, Tel: +39 069 722 3205; Fax: +39 069 722 3213; Email: vincenzo.barbera@aslromag.it.

procedures. CI-AKI is the third cause of renal failure acquired during hospitalization, after surgery and hypotension. Formerly the definition of AKI wasn't well defined due to poor knowledge of risk factors, pathogenesis and prevention strategies to reduce clinical manifestations especially in presence of predisposing conditions. The aforementioned items we'll describe based on the most recent knowledge and the last KDIGO guidelines.

## ACUTE KIDNEY INJURY*

***Jieun Kwak†, MD, and Shireen Hashmat‡, MD***
[1]Fellow in Neonatal-Perinatal Medicine, Department of Pediatrics
University of Southern California Medical Center,
Los Angeles County, CA, US
[2]Division of Pediatric Nephrology, Comer Children's Hospital, Chicago, IL, US

- Acute kidney injury is common in critically ill neonates hospitalized in the neonatal intensive care unit, and is associated with both short- and long-term increased risk for morbidity and mortality
- Diagnostic evaluation of acute kidney injury may include urine studies, serum laboratory studies, and imaging studies, depending on the clinical presentation
- Management of acute kidney injury is focused on: fluid management, electrolyte normalization, promotion of kidney perfusion, and blood pressure management

* The full version of this chapter can be found in *Essential Guide to Clinical Neonatology*, edited by Joseph R. Hageman, Alison Chu and Jeanette D. Hoenig, published by Nova Science Publishers, Inc, New York, 2016.

† Jkwak42@gmail.com.
‡ shashmat@peds.bsd.uchicago.edu.

# The Kidney and Acute Kidney Injury in HELLP Syndrome‡


***Sarah Novotny§, MD, MS, FACOG and Nicole M. Lee, MD, MPH, MS***

[1]Assistant Professor, Division of Maternal-Fetal Medicine
Department of Obstetrics and Gynecology
The University of Mississippi Medical Center
Jackson, MS, US
[2]Fellow, Maternal-Fetal Medicine,
Department of Obstetrics and Gynecology
The University of Mississippi Medical Center, Jackson, MS, US


Acute kidney injury (AKI), previously termed acute renal failure, is defined the abrupt loss of kidney function that can range from transient depression of renal function to irreversible renal disease and death. Over the last five decades, rates of AKI in pregnancy have decreased dramatically due largely to decreased rates of septic abortion and improvements in obstetric care. Today HELLP syndrome and severe forms of preeclampsia account for approximately 40% of all cases of AKI in pregnancy. However, despite the recent overall decrease in pregnancy-associated AKI, its occurrence in patients with HELLP syndrome has continued to range between 3-15% over multiple decades where renal injury in such patients can have a complex and lasting effect. Some investigators have reported that 30-50% of patients with acute renal failure (ARF) and HELLP syndrome require dialysis, and when patients develop AKI in HELLP syndrome, the perinatal mortality rate reaches 26%. Patients with pre-existing renal disease that develop HELLP syndrome have an even higher risk of perinatal mortality. Due to these risks, understanding renal injury in the setting of HELLP syndrome is of clinical importance for acute patient management as well as the prevention of long-term morbidity.

‡ The full version of this chapter can be found in *The 2015 Compendium for HELLP Syndrome: From Bench to Bedside*, edited James N. Martin, Jr., published by Nova Science Publishers, Inc, New York, 2015.

§ Email: snovotny@umc.edu

# ACUTE KIDNEY INJURY: CLASSIFICATION AND PROGNOSIS*

***Biruh Workeneh*†, *MD, FASN***
Division of Nephrology, Baylor College of Medicine

Acute kidney injury (AKI) is responsible for roughly 2 million deaths annually and is a major public health concern. [1] Fortunately, there has been tremendous progress in understanding the pathologic mechanisms, early detection, risk stratification and prognosis of AKI in the last decade. The impetus for revisiting AKI is because of the now established link between AKI and the development of chronic kidney disease (CKD). The traditional dogma taught to generations of physicians, which presumed that patients who suffered AKI fully recovered, is not universal. AKI-CKD is a spectrum and is indeed bidirectional; CKD is also a major risk factor for AKI and vice versa. [2] These revelations have resulted in a new era, reinventing our approach to the classification, detection and prevention of AKI. Parenthetically, the significance of the expanded role of electronic medical records and digitization in clinical practice cannot be underestimated and has allowed investigators, such as the ones we will discuss, to foster quality improvement in the field of AKI.

* The full version of this chapter can be found in *Essentials of Chronic Kidney Disease*, edited by Stephen Z. Fadem, published by Nova Science Publishers, Inc, New York, 2015.

† Corresponding author: Biruh Workeneh, MD, FASN; 6620 Main, Ste 11C; Houston, TX 77030; Ph: 713-798-8350; Fax: 713-798-3510.

# NGAL AS MARKER FOR PROGNOSIS OF ACUTE KIDNEY INJURY*

***Michael Haase*† *and Anja Haase-Fielitz***
Department of Nephrology, Hypertension, Diabetes and Endocrinology, Otto-von-Guericke University Magdeburg, Germany

Prognosis of a disease has a central role in clinical decision-making. A *prognostic biomarker* is a marker that provides information on the likely course and outcome of the disease. In a genomwide screening for novel renal biomarkers and proteomic follow-up experiments, neutrophil gelatinase-associated lipocalin (NGAL) was identified as the gene with the highest mRNA and protein levels in the kidney, urine, and plasma and with the earliest rise and peak after renal ischemia. The observed dose-effect response in numerous animal and human studies makes a favorable prognostic value for NGAL likely. The prognostic value of NGAL has now been investigated in several thousands of patients undergoing cardiac surgery, kidney transplantation, or critical illness. Five years after the initial meta-analysis, the overall value of NGAL for prognosis of acute kidney injury (AKI) and associated adverse outcomes across various patient populations remains essentially unchanged. The most frequently reported endpoints in biomarker studies on AKI prognosis are: AKI progression, requirement of renal replacement therapy (RRT), transition of AKI to chronic kidney disease (CKD), and mortality. This chapter condenses recent data on NGAL as marker for AKI prognosis.

* The full version of this chapter can be found in *Neutrophil Gelatinase-Associated Lipocalin: from Laboratory to Clinical Utility*, edited by Mina Hur and Salvatore Di Somma, published by Nova Science Publishers, Inc, New York, 2014.
† Correspondence: michael.haase@med.ovgu.de.

# NGAL: A Marker for Acute Kidney Injury*

*W. Frank Peacock*†*, MD, FACEP*
Emergency Medicine, Baylor College of Medicine,
Ben Taub General Hospital, Houston, Texas, US

Neutrophil gelatinase-associated lipocalin (NGAL), a member of the lipocalin family of proteins and secreted by kidney tubule cells at low levels, increases dramatically after ischemic, septic, or nephrotoxic renal injury.

Identifying acute kidney injury (AKI) early in its course could allow interventions preventing worsening renal function (WRF), thus the use of NGAL to detect early AKI may be of considerable clinical importance. The use of NGAL as a marker of AKI has been specifically evaluated in the emergency department (ED), a population with uncharacterized illness and whose kidney injury is often evolving.

Data in literature demonstrated that the assessment of patient's initial blood NGAL when admitted to hospital from ED improved the initial clinical diagnosis of AKI, moreover NGAL assessment coupled with the ED physician's clinical judgment may prove useful in deciding the appro-priate strategies for patients at risk for the development of AKI.

Finally, presentation NGAL > 400 ng/mL had the highest predictive value for in-hospital patient's mortality of all the evaluated predictive parameters.

* The full version of this chapter can be found in *Neutrophil Gelatinase-Associated Lipocalin: from Laboratory to Clinical Utility*, edited by Mina Hur and Salvatore Di Somma, published by Nova Science Publishers, Inc, New York, 2014.

† Correspondence: W. Frank Peacock. E-mail: Frankpeacock@gmail.com.

# ACUTE KIDNEY INJURY IN SEPSIS*

***Marcelo Rodrigues Bacci*†, *MD***
Assistant Professor- General Practice Department-
Faculdade de Medicina do ABC
(ABC Medical School)- São Paulo- Brazil

Sepsis and acute kidney injury (AKI) are two of the main causes of hospitalization in intensive care units (ICU) and account for a large proportion of deaths in these units in spite of continuous intense investigation at different levels. Sepsis is one of the leading cause of AKI. Understanding its pathophysiology was difficult in the past because of lack of data from study of kidney biopsies. Therefore, the so called "Acute Tubular Necrosis" did not fit in this scenario as sepsis-induced AKI is a major hemodynamic situation with an increase in blood flow and a decrease in filtration pressure. Also, there are non-hemodynamic factors that play an important role in sepsis- induced AKI. The cytokines like interleukin-6, interleukin-1, tumor necrosis factor-alpha act as potential stimulators of apoptosis, leukocyte activation and necrosis. Treatment of Sepsis-induced AKI is directed at controlling the arterial pressure, managing glycemia and using appropriate antimicrobial therapy. Specific substances to stop the process of AKI are not available 1 yet for human usage. Dialysis methods should be chosen based on patients' needs.

* The full version of this chapter can be found in *Sepsis: Diagnosis, Management and Health Outcomes*, edited by Nancy Khardori, published by Nova Science Publishers, Inc, New York, 2014.

† Email: mrbacci@yahoo.com

# ACUTE KIDNEY INJURY ON CHRONIC KIDNEY DISEASE - THE RAINBOW SYNDROME OF TOO MANY COLORS: A MAYO CLINIC HEALTH SYSTEM CASE SERIES REPORT*

*Macaulay Amechi Onuigbo, M.D., M.Sc., F.W.A.C.P., F.A.S.N., M.B.A.*[1,2,†] *and Ngozi Janet Achebe, M.D.*[3]

[1]Mayo Clinic College of Medicine, Rochester, MN, USA

[2]Department of Nephrology, Mayo Clinic Health System, Eau Claire, WI, USA

[3]Capital Medical Center, Olympia, WA, USA

Whereas nephrologists and physicians are conversant with the common diagnosis of acute kidney injury (AKI) on chronic kidney disease (CKD), however, the common consensus is that this is usually transient, with typical expected recovery of renal function in most instances. Nevertheless, both anecdotal as well as objective evidence support the contrary conception that quite often, there is much less renal recovery following these AKI on CKD events. Furthermore, there is increasing new evidence in the literature that AKI not only leads to and propagates CKD, but that AKI could directly lead to irreversible ESRD and the need for permanent renal replacement therapy. In this chapter, we describe some cases representing the various patterns of renal outcomes following AKI on CKD. We show that renal outcomes following AKI on CKD is a spectrum of a continuum from quick complete recovery of a priori renal functional status, through various degrees of partial renal functional recovery, to the rapid and unpredictable precipitate progression to acute yet irreversible ESRD in one continuum of time without any renal recovery ever taking place, with such AKI-ESRD translations sometimes occurring very rapidly over only days to weeks. The later phenomenon is the syndrome of rapid onset end-stage renal disease (SORO-ESRD), a previously unrecognized syndrome which we first described in the journal *Renal Failure* in 2010. Undeniably, the variable renal outcomes that could follow AKI on

* The full version of this chapter can be found in *ACE Inhibitors: Medical Uses, Mechanisms of Action, Potential Adverse Effects and Related Topics. Volume 1*, edited by Macaulay Amechi Onuigbo, published by Nova Science Publishers, Inc, New York, 2013.

† E-mail: onuigbo.macaulay@mayo.edu.

CKD events could indeed best be described as the several colors of the rainbow. We conclude this chapter by acknowledging the global AKI, CKD and ESRD pandemics. We have called for stronger attention to be paid to the prevention of AKI through the increased awareness of providers of the potential for drug-related nephrotoxicities, more pharmacovigilance and an enhanced application of the principles of renoprevention, a paradigm we first reported in 2009 that involves the deliberate protocolizedprevention or rapid correction of peri-operative hypotension, and the deliberate pre-emptive withdrawal or avoidance of all potential nephrotoxic exposures in the peri-operative period and during concurrent serious illness. Finally, in this chapter, we have again re-introduced the concept of 'triple whammy', first described by Thomas in 2000, the association of AKI with the concurrent use of combination, diuretics, ACEIs/ARBs and NSAIDs. Furthermore, we have described in another chapter of this book, in great detail, a related new syndrome, that we dubbed 'quadruple whammy', that we first described in a commentary published in the British Medical Journal in the Spring of 2013.

## PREVENTION OF ACUTE KIDNEY INJURY IN CRITICALLY ILL PATIENTS*

***Marlies Ostermann***†

King's College London, Guy's and St. Thomas' Hospital, London, United Kingdom

Acute kidney injury is associated with significant short and long-term complications and increased mortality. The key elements of primary and secondary prevention are prompt recognition of the patients at risk, timely goal directed resuscitation of the circulation with fluids and vasoactive drugs, and avoidance of additional renal damage. A mean arterial pressure ≥65 mmHg should be aimed for but higher targets may be necessary in patients with severe sepsis / septic shock and/or pre-existing chronic hypertension. There is

* The full version of this chapter can be found in *Renal Failure: Prevention, Causes and Treatment*, edited by Colin Andrew Hutchison, published by Nova Science Publishers, Inc, New York, 2013.

† E-mail: Marlies.Ostermann@gstt.nhs.uk.

no role for diuretics, thyroxine, statins, erythropoietin, natriuretic peptide, aprotinine, activated protein C, tight glucose control, steroids or calcium channel blockers to prevent AKI in critically ill patients. If possible, nephrotoxic drugs should be discontinued. Strategies for prevention of AKI across a range of different groups are discussed, including patients with cardiac disease, liver cirrhosis, tumour lysis syndrome, rhabdomyolysis and intra-abdominal hypertension.

# ACUTE KIDNEY INJURY*

## *Atul Sajgure[1] and Devasmita Choudhury[2]*

[1]Consultant Nephrologist, Sahyadri Specialty Hospital, Pune, Maharastra, India

[2]Associate Professor Medicine, UTSouthwestern Medical School, Director In-Center and Home Dialysis, VA North Texas Healthcare System, Dallas VA Medical Center, Dallas TX, USA

Acute Kidney Injury (AKI) previously termed acute renal failure is a common, often complex clinical process which can be devastating. Broadly defined as a rapid decline in glomerular filtration rate (i.e., over hours and weeks), AKI is potentially reversible. AKI can occur in patients with normal kidney function or in those with underlying chronic kidney disease. With early detection, recovery from AKI frequently occurs sooner with extrinsic causes of functional renal loss such as pre-renal processes or post renal obstruction. Intrinsic renal processes often result in more prolonged renal injury and require renal support. While injury, inflammation or obstruction of any of the intrinsic renal structures can result in and present as acute kidney injury, the most common presentation is acute ischemic, nephrotoxic or sepsis related acute kidney injury and tubular necrosis. Reported incidences of AKI have varied based on non-uniform clinical definitions precluding comparison and validation of clinical outcomes. Approximately 5% of hospitalized patients and up to 50% of all intensive care unit (ICU) patients are diagnosed with AKI. Current evidence suggests that despite major advances in the treatment

* The full version of this chapter can be found in *Nephropathy: Diagnosis and Treatment*, edited by Stephen Fava, published by Nova Science Publishers, Inc, New York, 2012.

of AKI, long-term morbidity is a frequent complication with 5-year patient survival estimates of 65 and 70%. The presence of AKI independently predicts the risk of death. Mortality with AKI in the hospital is 10 times greater than those hospitalized without AKI, particularly when renal support is necessary. For critically ill patients with multi-organ failure, reported mortality ranges from 50-80%. Continued risk for increased morbidity and mortality has prompted greater scrutiny of the definition, pathobiology and management of AKI which will be targets for discussion in this chapter.

## Acute Kidney Injury: Assessment of Kidney Function and Damage*

*Wonngarm Kittanamongkolchai*†*, Napat Leeaphorn, Pongsathorn Kue-A-Pai and Wisit Cheungpasitporn*

Department of Internal Medicine, Bassett Medical Center, Cooperstown, New York, US

Acute kidney injury (AKI) is characterized by a rapid decline in glomerular filtration rate (GFR) over hours to days that results in the retention of urea and other nitrogenous waste products normally cleared by the kidneys. It is associated with a 25% to 80% risk of in-hospital death and has been rising in the incidence over the past several decades. The RIFLE and AKIN criteria have greatest utility in epidemiologic studies. However, these definitions may be problematic when applied to patients at bedside because the baseline creatinine may be unknown. The creatinine (Cr) level may not perfectly reflect the severity of kidney injury because serum Cr is altered by age, sex, muscle mass, nutritional status, and medications. The novel biomarkers, such as Kidney injury molecule-1 (KIM-1) and Neutrophil gelatinase associated lipocalin (NGAL), are promising in the diagnosis of intrinsic AKI and may permit development of a new paradigm for classifying AKI in the future.

* The full version of this chapter can be found in *Creatinine: Production, Diagnostic Uses and Role in Renal Disease*, edited by Ivan H. Perkins and Catherine M. Chapman, published by Nova Science Publishers, Inc, New York, 2012.

† Email: wonngarm.kittanamongkolchai@bassett.org

# Index

## D



## E

## F



## G



## H



## I

## J



## K



## L



## M

## N



## O



## P



## Q



## R

## S



## T



## U

## V



## W